Women OVER 40 CAN'T LOSE WEIGHT

GABRIELLE O'HARE

First published in paperback by
Michael Terence Publishing in 2022
www.mtp.agency

ISBN 9781800944046

Michael Terence
Publishing

For Tim

With heartfelt thanks for your unconditional love and constant encouragement to follow my dreams.

CONTENTS

INTRODUCTION

Why do women over 40 find it so hard to lose weight? This is something I've been asking myself for years, and this book finally answers this perplexing question.

Most diets are created with little understanding or empathy for how middle-aged women experience dieting. They tell us what we should and shouldn't eat but don't explain why we simply can't cope with feeling hungry and deprived. Women face a complex set of problems that intensify as we approach menopause. Plus, we've been conditioned to believe that our bodies will change, whether we like it or not, and that there is little we can do about it.

Yet we don't want to lose control over our bodies. Not understanding why our weight and shape are changing is frightening and overwhelming. For many, this is far more than an aesthetic concern. If we can't regain control over our weight, what does that mean for the future?

Approaching middle age is daunting in its own right, and women have the spectre of menopause to contend with. We're not ready to fade into the background and compromise on living our lives. We want energy and drive, and to feel good about ourselves. But for many, this is a time when self-confidence plummets, often due to how our bodies have changed.

Whilst we live in an age where body positivity and physical inclusivity is rightly celebrated, this is about something different. Our bodies are changing into something we don't recognise. We don't understand why or know what to do about it. So, we turn to dieting in the hope we can lose weight and rediscover a body we're more familiar with. But despite our best intentions, attempts to diet are short-lived.

Before long, cravings overpower us again. We run out of time and energy to make healthy meals and order takeaways even when our fridges are full. Our families insist we buy junk that we can't resist, and we cave in to pressure to abandon our diets when we eat with friends and family. Sugar is our lifeline when we're running on empty, and we feel like we deserve every treat that passes our lips. It's a lonely battle.

Not being able to lose weight is less about age and willpower and more about how lifestyles and hormones prevent us from making the consistent changes that bring results. Until now, you might have blamed yourself for failing, for being lazy and greedy. But you're about to learn that thousands of other women are in the same boat and have experienced similar frustrations.

This book tackles weight loss from an entirely new perspective. It's not a new, miracle diet; instead, it highlights six major blockers that affect how we eat and prevent us from sticking with a diet long enough for it to work. Nothing weird happens to women after 40 that prevents them from losing weight. From my experience, it's only harder because our lives have become harder. By this age, we've probably spent decades neglecting ourselves while we've focused on other things. And, like most of the population, we've lost our connection with the importance of real food.

However, before you can lose weight this time, you must first uncover why you have struggled in the past, and this book will help you do that. Until then, no diet will work because the same blockers will come up repeatedly, whichever approach you try.

To lose weight at this age means more than cutting calories and working out. That might have worked in our 20s and 30s, but now we must add a few other changes into the mix. Menopause has a bearing on weight, affecting hormones and eating patterns. The same issues that cause us to gain weight also sap energy levels, flatten moods and erode motivation. The advice in this book will address all these factors, putting you back in control of your body. But this isn't just a book about losing weight. The changes that I recommend you make to your lifestyle will give you more energy; they'll make you feel stronger, calmer, able to think clearly and be more in control of your life. This is vastly more important than what you weigh.

It's my absolute belief that if every woman over the age of 40 stayed strong, healthy, and energetic, the world would be a better place. But it's an uphill battle because society isn't kind to women over a certain age. Our workloads are relentless, and despite giving so much of ourselves to others, we feel invisible and ignored. The wisdom and value we still have to offer are not willingly accepted, and we have to fight to stay relevant. Menopause turns the screw even tighter with symptoms which affect every aspect of our lives, leaving us feeling overwhelmed, exhausted, and isolated. Surely, we cannot accept that it's OK for half the population to struggle for the second half of their lives.

Women need better access to HRT, employers need better policies to support us through menopause, and we need better representation of older women in the media. Fortunately, all of this is slowly changing for the better, but we must also be part of this change by taking better care of ourselves and recognising and honouring our own value. We can't criticise society for ignoring us if we keep putting ourselves last all the time.

We've spent long enough prioritising others and it's time to turn our attention to ourselves. This is our time. We don't need to fade quietly into the background of other people's lives. Instead, if we work at our health and well-being we can emerge like a butterfly from its chrysalis, feeling invigorated and excited about what's to come. Because the stronger we are and the better we feel, the more we can live to our full potential and make the second half of our lives as good, or even better than the first.

Over the past couple of years as a Personal Trainer, I've met an incredible group of women who have inspired me every day with their unique capacity to love and care for others. Every woman who came to me for support wanted the same thing, to feel better in herself. Some had recovered from serious illnesses; others had to deal with frightening diagnoses that highlighted the importance of their health. Others wanted to stay healthy for their families, develop their careers, find the stamina to start new businesses or embark on an active retirement. They wanted the energy and confidence to live a life in which they could keep giving, stay sane and have fun, which they absolutely deserved. And I hope I've been able to help them achieve that.

In return, by trusting me to support them, they've given me powerful insights into the reasons behind their struggles. When we are vulnerable and open about what we find challenging, we uncover the things we share. When we discover we aren't alone in our struggles, we find ways to support each other and help each other succeed.

My wish for you is that this book shines a light on the things that are holding you back and gives you the tools to cut through the complexities of real life, so you can reclaim your right to feel amazing.

• PART ONE •

THE REAL REASONS YOU CAN'T STICK TO A DIET

Why can't we stick to diets? In my experience, most people manage a concerted effort that lasts two or maybe three weeks. Something knocks us off track, and going hungry or depriving ourselves of our favourite foods feels unbearable, and we can't cope with the extra effort required to keep going. Most diets are abandoned before the results show, and even if we lose a few pounds, it comes back faster than it came off.

Women are hard on themselves when they fail. I hear so many women blaming themselves for being lazy when they are anything but. We also blame hormones or slow metabolism, or imagine we have some mysterious condition that means we'll never be able to lose weight. In those situations, we think we can't do anything about it and are destined to helplessly watch our waistlines expand.

What really holds us back is rarely acknowledged or discussed. Constant demands placed on us by family, society's expectations of women, and even our environment hugely impact what we eat. Eating habits are tightly woven into every part of our lives, and decisions about what and when we eat are influenced by many things outside ourselves. As the demands on our time increase, we have to cut corners, so we turn to convenience food. But that doesn't answer the problem of why we're gaining weight. The question then is not so much why can't we stick to a diet, but why can't we stop eating?

I love food and eating, but am tormented by the need to feel full and satisfied. To find something to eat that switches off cravings and leaves me in peace. Resisting the urge to eat is incredibly hard. You're locked in constant negotiation with a little voice in your head telling you to just have one more. You're always thinking about food, what you're going to eat next, and find it impossible to concentrate on other things.

Being responsible for organising and cooking family meals makes it even harder to escape from obsessing about food. We have to think about food when we're not hungry. Planning the shopping, checking cupboards for supplies, getting things out of the freezer and cooking meals. The rest of the family doesn't need to bother with all this. As soon as they're hungry and want to eat, it's all ready and waiting.

As I coached more and more women, I realised we all shared similar problems. Eventually, clear patterns emerged, and I identified six distinct issues that make it impossible for us to stick with a diet.

Self-neglect. Putting the needs of families and careers first and allowing our own needs to take a back seat.

Stress. Suffering from chronic stress, which affects hormones, fat accumulation and eating habits.

Menopause. Suffering from direct and indirect symptoms that affect weight gain, fat distribution, eating habits and cravings.

An unhealthy relationship with food. Using food as a coping mechanism and forming other unhealthy eating habits.

Sabotage. Pressure and resistance from others when we try to eat better.

Advertisers dream. Being inadvertently influenced by food marketing for ultra-processed foods which affects appetite and cravings.

In the following chapters, I detail each of these to help you identify your biggest diet blockers. I promise that once you understand your weaknesses, learning to overcome the challenges that hold you back will give you better results than any new diet.

Self-Neglect

Self-neglect isn't a wilful disregard for our health. Instead, it's symptomatic of women's many roles, society's expectations of us, and the pressure we place on ourselves. The transition from single and carefree happens slowly, and with every achievement from the list of goals we've been aiming for, we gradually get squeezed out of our own lives by the pressure of keeping each plate spinning.

One of the things that's struck me most about the women I've trained is how much they care about what they do, but there's a price for this integrity. We have an inbuilt desire to play each of our roles to the best of our ability. To be a dutiful daughter, the perfect wife, the doting mum, a reliable friend, an active community member, a conscientious worker, and a caring boss. Alongside each of these personas, we're running homes, stocking cupboards, and striving for domestic order.

Women are society's givers and carers. We're brilliant organisers, and we love feeling needed. We constantly worry about the important people in our lives, trying to anticipate what they need and doing our utmost to ensure they get it. But in doing so, we sacrifice what we need. We struggle with the notion of putting ourselves first because society has conditioned us not to be selfish. At home, even if we get help from partners, we still get a raw deal. We do more than our fair share of chores and are more likely to carry the mental load of remembering everything and checking things get done.

At work, we're more likely than men to experience gendered ageism, which increases the pressure on us to stay relevant. And menopause can have a profound effect on performance at work. Support from employers is often absent, so we have no option other than to peddle even harder to keep up, but that's not always enough. I've seen far too many harried forty-somethings dashing from one meeting to the next, surviving on coffee and chocolate. They're overloaded with work, thanks to their decades of experience, and face constant firefighting whilst being terrified of saying no to their managers.

As children grow up, parental roles change. Teenagers challenge us in ways we never expected and leave us feeling out of our depth. Several women have told me they often feel trapped at home now their kids are older. When they were little, we accepted we had to look after them 24/7 and were rewarded with endless cuddles and cute smiles. Now we sit around in case they emerge from dark bedrooms, hopeful of a conversation. They probably wouldn't notice if we went out, but we can't seem to cut loose and instead wait patiently for any signs that show they still love us.

Our kids might not need us, but our parents do. This is the age where we begin to worry about their health and face up to the inevitable. Daughters and daughters-in-law take on caring roles, which can last years. Several of my clients do regular overnight stays with parents or in-laws just so they can remain in their own homes. I lost my dad during lockdown, and nothing prepares you for how the loss of a parent changes your identity.

The endless list of physical tasks combined with the mental load of remembering, organising, worrying and anticipating is exhausting. There are only twenty-four hours in a day, and we become so stretched we leave no time for ourselves.

Case studies

Jo was in her mid-40s and clinically obese. Her knees troubled her so much that she struggled to keep up with the kids and desperately wanted to lose weight. She was the primary earner and worked full-time. Because her husband found it hard to deal with the kids, she did most of the childcare. Working from home allowed her to do the school pick-up and make dinner, but this meant going back on her laptop when they'd gone to bed and frequently working until the early hours. Meals came out of the freezer, and she constantly snacked during the day because she didn't have time to stop. Weekends were precious family time. She knew there were far too many treats and meals out, but this was the only time she got to relax, and she felt she deserved it.

Kerry was gaining weight as she went through menopause. She was in her early 50s and had three teenagers at home. She loved watching them blossoming into adults but couldn't help comparing herself to them. She increasingly felt her age and was becoming self-conscious about her weight. Despite working part-time, she was constantly on the go, doing housework and cooking. Evenings were spent dropping kids off at various places before picking them up again, so she rarely sat down until late into the evening. Making meals the family enjoyed was important to her, but a lot of processed food had crept in over the years. Now and again, she tried to eat healthier and take regular walks, which she did enjoy, but she could never keep it up for long because she didn't have time. She relied too heavily on snacks to keep her energy up, and whenever she got a minute, she needed a sit down more than a workout.

Amna worked full-time in her own business. Every weekend her young granddaughter slept over so her daughter could have a night off. Amna needed to lose weight and was diabetic. A few years earlier, she damaged her knee in a car crash, and walking was painful. Knowing losing weight would help, she did a weekly PT session, but her weight stayed the same. Constantly putting her work and daughter first left her exhausted. She never had a minute to herself and started to resent that no one seemed to care how she felt. Convenience food and sugary snacks kept her going. She knew she wasn't eating properly but simply couldn't find the energy or motivation to cook. The extra calories meant her weight stayed the same, despite exercising. She was desperate to change but was at her limit. She was at a loss to know how to reduce her responsibilities without letting down the people she loved.

How self-neglect affects your weight

These are real examples of prioritising others to the extent we neglect ourselves. Our attention is firmly focused on everyone and everything except us. We become highly attuned and attentive to others and watch vigilantly for signs that things are off, so we can swiftly catch problems before they take hold, to keep things running smoothly.

Yet, as we've become hypersensitive to others, we've stopped listening to ourselves and barely register our own needs. We tell colleagues they need a break, but we won't take one. We let families off the hook with chores, but we end up doing them. One client fed her beloved dog a premium diet and faithfully followed the vet's advice that he only eat once a day, but constantly snacked herself.

We want the best for everyone but have put our needs on hold for so long, we've forgotten how to take care of ourselves. Over the years, this neglect gradually builds up, and it shows in our weight, our energy levels and eventually our mood.

Making meals others want. This is a typical pattern where we allow others' eating preferences to take priority over our own. We ask our families what they want for dinner, and once we've taken the order, we cook it. Making food for loved ones is just another way we express love for them. Yet kids rarely want broccoli and meat. We pureed organic vegetables when we weaned them as infants, but now we're emptying packets of frozen food onto oven trays. Clients sometimes tell me their husbands and kids can eat what they want without putting on weight, but they can't. Instinctively we know we should be eating differently but reversing these habits is another chore we don't have time for.

No time to eat properly. Days are hectic from the minute we get up, and taking time to sit down for meals has become a luxury. If you're lucky, breakfast is eaten on the go, and you'll eat lunch at your desk. But many don't have time to stop for meals. When you're constantly on the go, you're more likely to skip meals and rely on snacks to keep your energy up. If you've not had chance to eat properly all day, you end up ravenous later. It might seem like you've barely eaten, but the constant eating adds up to more calories than you realise, and you're still more likely to overeat in the evening.

Relying on convenience food. When time is at a premium, we must find the most efficient ways to get everything done. Gradually we've drifted towards ready-made convenience foods. It saves time, and no one complains. Why bother preparing a packed lunch for work when you can nip into a shop for something someone else has made? Retailers make mealtimes super easy for us, but there's a price. We're more likely to overeat processed foods, and tempted by offers, we buy and eat way more than we need.

No energy. Being constantly at the beck and call of others is physically and mentally draining. When our only option is to crack on, sugar and caffeine give us a temporary lift. At the end of a busy day, we've not got the energy to make homemade dinners or go out for a run.

Using treats as rewards. Humans seek rewards for their efforts, our brains are wired that way. Without rewards, drive and motivation disappear, and we wouldn't get things done. We live in a society where food and alcohol are advertised as alluring treats, and they are never more than an arm's reach from us. They fit perfectly into hectic lives because no effort is required to pop the cork from a bottle of fizz or peel back a plastic lid to reveal a decadent dessert. We work so hard that we have no problem justifying these indulgences. And can you blame us? But the calories still add up.

Stress

Stress is the emotional consequence of ignoring our needs. Decades of being always on leave us overstimulated, like hyperactive kids who've overdosed on sugar at a birthday party. But the more demands we accumulate, the harder it is to stay on top of everything.

It's not just the sheer volume of tasks that are the problem. It's the constant pressure of having them on our minds. Women often suffer from overactive minds. We worry about getting everything done on time, create elaborate backup plans in case things don't go to plan and rack our brains to make sure we've not forgotten anything. We're also prone to catastrophising, creating imaginary worst-case scenarios that leave us paralysed with fear about things that will never happen. Have you ever noticed how hot your phone becomes when you use it too long? That's the heat generated by internal processors drawing energy from the battery. It's precisely the same with our brains. Endless mental wrangling uses energy - and lots of it, leaving us drained and frazzled.

In the same way exhausted toddlers fight bedtime, we continue the same pattern. In our quest to keep ploughing through to-do lists, we ignore that diminutive voice pleading with us to slow down. Our bodies are designed to switch between two modes: rest and recovery and fight or flight. When faced with immediate pressure, we switch into fight or flight mode, a state of high alert characterised by a sharp mind and being pumped full of energy. When the sh*t hits the fan, we step into our most capable and powerful selves, and it feels amazing when we nail challenging situations.

As alluring as it feels, we're not designed to stay like this. Once the drama is over, we're supposed to flip back into rest and recovery mode; to chill out and have some fun. Now the need to be on high alert has passed, our bodies resume their normal duty of keeping vital processes ticking over, while we take things easy.

Except we don't allow ourselves to rest and recover. In fact, we're terrible at it, but we don't think we have a choice. I'm often asked for advice on how to make diets more effective or what sort of exercise is best for weight loss. Women listen when I answer these questions, but if I tell them they need to reduce the stress they're under, they don't want to know. Tackling stress pushes us into the uncomfortable territory of having to say no, letting people down and even admitting defeat. All these things go against our deepest values and identities. But refusing to slow down will eventually catch up on us. We think this is just a battle of will, but in reality, stress is slowly but surely attacking our bodies, and one way it does this, is by increasing levels of abdominal fat.

Client case study

Beth was in her mid-fifties and wanted to drop a couple of dress sizes. She trained with me twice a week, and we created a solid plan for her diet. She subscribed to a pre-planned meal delivery service, which had a calorie-counted range, so she could easily track her calories. Beth had everything going for her to make losing weight straightforward. Yet over the 6 months we trained together, she lost and put on the same 3-4lb and never hit her goal.

Beth had a considerable amount of stress in her life. Work was demanding, and her youngest son was leaving for university in a few months. She knew this was the beginning of her life as an empty nester and didn't know how to fill the gap he would leave. Her parents were getting older, and she constantly worried about them, feeling guilty that she wasn't there for them as much as she would have liked. Working from home during lockdown meant long hours in front of her computer, and she worked late into the evening. Unsurprisingly, she struggled to switch off and didn't sleep well most nights.

Beth was adding more stress into her life in her quest to lose weight. To fit workouts into her already hectic schedule, she trained at 7am, often after poor sleep and already anticipating problems stacking up in her inbox. Slowly and silently, stress was accumulating on all fronts. Staying on top of everything took more effort than it used to, and being able to switch off and enjoy herself was becoming increasingly elusive.

Yet, thriving under pressure was part of Beth's identity. She was a high achiever and had spent decades working in an industry where stress was part of the job description, so she was blind to how much it was building up. With previous diets, she got results because she was always prepared to do more and work harder, but that approach wasn't working this time. It's a fine line between thriving on stress and getting worn down by it. At this time of her life, it was wearing her down and preventing her from hitting her goal.

Chronic (constant) stress

In addition to coping with strenuous workloads, so many everyday situations trigger stress that we don't realise how much we are under. At this stage of our lives, it's common for many relationships to shift, often out of our control. Coping with teenagers is totally different to managing toddler tantrums. Romantic and personal relationships change, and not always for the better, and we may even take on new roles as carers. Dealing with difficult colleagues or toxic friendships is obviously stressful, and another problem is feeling drained by too much interpersonal contact. Several women I've recently spoken to mentioned experiencing this. They were unsure if it was a post-lockdown phenomenon or more to do with their hormones. Either way, it affected their behaviour to the extent of avoiding social situations because they found them too draining.

Smartphone use also triggers a stress response, and given how frequently we interact with them, they have the potential to significantly add to our stress load. These are some of the ways your phone can give you stress:

- Needing to instantly respond to notifications on your phone
- Being compelled to keep checking social media for likes, comments and messages
- Feelings of inadequacy when viewing social content
- Worrying about what people think of your posts

Being constantly exposed to negative news is another trigger. Living under a cloud of doom and gloom induces fearful thoughts and creates extra worries about how situations we can't control might affect our own lives.

As a result, many people now suffer from chronic stress, meaning they are constantly exposed to low-level stress, which elevates stress hormones.

How stress makes us fat

Elevated stress hormones affect the way we store fat. Most people think body fat is related to how much we eat, but it's not that simple. Stress releases a hormone called cortisol. Constant stress elevates levels of this hormone and is known to increase abdominal fat.[1] If you're gaining extra fat around your middle and don't understand why, this could be the reason.

Abdominal fat can be very hard to shift. Diet and exercise aren't always effective at dealing with it because cutting calories too low and over-exercising stress the body even more. Stress can have such a powerful effect on body fat that the advice for people who need to lose weight but are under excessive stress, is to prioritise reducing stress over any other intervention.

In addition to creating hormone imbalances that influence fat storage, stress also affects other behaviours around food. At the end of a stressful day, have you noticed how hard it is to decide what to make for dinner or find the motivation to make a healthy meal from scratch? Chronic stress leaves us feeling overwhelmed and reduces our decision-making capacity. In these situations, we subconsciously default to the easiest options, like ordering a takeaway or getting something out of the freezer. Whilst this seems like a reasonable solution, these foods are often high in calories and low in nutrition.

Chronic stress is linked to poor sleep. If we engage in cortisol-stimulating activities like scrolling on our phones or working until late, we don't wind down and can't drop off. Even after one bad night, we're more likely to overeat, make poorer food choices and rely on sugar and caffeine to keep us going.[2]

Many people are aware that they eat when stressed. Have you ever felt upset and walked straight into the kitchen looking for food? Or found yourself struggling with a task and stopped to eat something instead? Challenging situations create uncomfortable sensations in the body, and snacking temporarily distracts us from them. This works so effectively that it soon becomes a deeply ingrained habit, and we find ourselves eating all day in response to the stress we're under.

Stress and overwhelm leave us feeling down. Food high in sugar, fat and refined flours are known to light up the dopamine receptors in the brain to give us an instant hit of pleasure. Eating something good is an easy way to cheer ourselves up, but the types of food we crave have hundreds of calories and trigger sugar crashes and cravings.

Some people manage to be 'good' during the week but undo everything at the weekend. Stress accumulates over time, leaving us desperate for a release when we can finally relax. Overeating comfort food and binge drinking at the weekend is often a response to hgh stress levels during the week.

Other stress symptoms

Stress is a natural part of our lives, and we'll always have some to deal with, but it's important not to let it get out of control. Pay attention to symptoms which suggest it may be affecting your well-being.

- Feeling constantly overwhelmed
- Being forgetful and finding it difficult to concentrate
- Experiencing incessant mental chatter
- Suffering from fearful and negative thoughts

- Disturbed sleep or inability to fall asleep easily
- Unable to switch off, even during the evening or at weekends
- Fighting the urge to relax by looking for things that keep you busy
- Unable to handle difficult situations that are normal in everyday life and overreacting by getting angry and upset
- Feeling tired and run down and suffering from regular coughs and colds
- Regularly experiencing a low mood or being irritable and snappy

Physical stress symptoms

Constantly elevated hormones caused by chronic stress can also cause serious physical symptoms, which affect health:

- Headaches and dizziness
- Muscle tension and pain
- Stomach and digestive problems
- Chest pains and heart palpitations
- High blood pressure
- Panic attacks
- Low libido
- Skin and hair problems

It's essential to tackle stress rather than ignore it. If you are suffering from any of the above, visit your GP to rule out other underlying causes and get support to bring stress under control.

Menopause

Just as life seems to reach its peak intensity, menopause shows up and turns the screw. We knew about middle-aged spread long before it affected us. For decades, we've been told that when we reach menopause, we have no choice but to accept this inevitable consequence of female ageing. This assumption always infuriated me, and I refused to believe it was true. But fortunately, whilst weight gain during menopause is common, it's not inevitable, and losing weight during this stage of your life is possible.

Perimenopause most often starts in women aged 40 to 44. Officially you reach menopause twelve months after your last period, and the average age for this is 51. According to the NHS, most symptoms continue for four years from your final period, while 1 in 10 women experience symptoms for up to twelve years.[3]

Many women experience symptoms well before they are officially menopausal. The complete list of symptoms is long and ranges from sleepless nights and low mood to itchy skin, heart palpitations, and brain fog. Yet, many women don't realise they are experiencing perimenopause because their periods are regular, and they aren't having well-known symptoms like hot flashes. The slow decline of hormones means many symptoms appear gradually. One client, in her mid-forties, often ended up in tears because she just couldn't get her act together. Instead of recognising early symptoms, we're more likely to blame ourselves for not being on our A-game.

Early signs include feeling more anxious and overwhelmed and being less able to cope than usual. Low mood is another, along with a sense life generally feels a little less bright. Motivation can drop, and we can't be bothered to put as much effort into things we used to enjoy. I used to love cooking for my family but suddenly became increasingly resentful about being stuck in the kitchen. Other women have noticed having less tolerance for feeling uncomfortable. A regular runner gave up because she couldn't stand the thought of feeling sweaty or breathless. Others become irritated by clothes, shoes or even underwear that weren't comfortable. Even being slightly hungry feels intolerable. By the time the penny drops that we're in perimenopause, we might have been coping with these symptoms for years.

The truth about menopause and middle-aged spread

Middle-age spread is caused by the combination of becoming less active and losing muscle mass. Muscle is active tissue, which means it burns calories. The more muscle we have, the more calories we burn. If we allow muscles to waste away but eat the same amount, we gradually put on weight.

A typical middle-aged body is not just a thicker waist. Arms and legs get thinner, bums get flatter, and shoulders become rounder. This is the effect of muscle wastage and poor posture. From around 30, we lose 5% of our muscle mass each decade.[4] Then, for several years after menopause, we lose muscle at a faster rate than at any other time of our life. Unless we do exercises that actively protect muscles, we could lose at least 15% of our total muscle mass between the ages of 30 and 60.[5]

Stress hormones, menopause and abdominal fat

Around menopause, stress has an even more significant impact on weight because of a new connection between oestrogen production and stress hormones. We still need oestrogen after the ovaries stop producing it, so our body has two other sources. Fat can make a weak source of oestrogen, so we lay down more body fat to increase its supply. Adrenal glands also start producing oestrogen, although their primary role is to produce stress hormones.

However, chronic stress plays havoc with this process because it forces the adrenals to default to their primary function of producing stress hormones, thus ceasing oestrogen production. To compensate for the shortfall, we lay down even more abdominal fat. In a double whammy, chronic stress raises cortisol levels, which further increases belly fat. This is how stress makes us fat and why it can worsen during menopause.

Menopause cruelly arrives at a time when we encounter many new stressors which are out of our control. When we need to be able to handle stress more than ever, menopause symptoms exacerbate it and reduce our ability to cope. This leaves us at greater risk of suffering from the many health risks associated with chronic stress, and our quality of life can suffer enormously. You can't understand why you can't cope with things you've been managing for years and can even be embarrassed and ashamed by how you feel. This can have life-changing consequences.

Many women are forced to take drastic action when holding down their job becomes too much. In one survey of 4,000 menopausal women, 50% resigned or took early retirement because of their perimenopause or menopause.[(6)] Unless you realise hormones are to blame, this can be a very bewildering, challenging, and lonely time.

How menopause symptoms affect your eating habits

It's not just hormonal changes that affect our fat levels. Many menopause symptoms have a knock-on effect on how we eat.

Poor sleep

Disturbed sleep is one of the most well-known menopause symptoms. Heightened stress and anxiety make it impossible to switch off before bed, so falling asleep can take ages. Hot flashes can wake you, and a full-blown hot sweat can soak you and your bedding to the extent you need to change the sheets. Falling back to sleep after such a distressing episode can take hours.

Poor sleep is linked to weight gain. It's a well-known fact that when we don't get enough sleep, we eat more calories and make less-healthy food choices the next day. When we wake up exhausted, we turn to coffee and sugar to boost energy. Overdoing the caffeine can compound the problem, making it harder to switch off and fall asleep at bedtime, creating a vicious cycle.

Mood & motivation, pleasure & cravings

Menopause can affect mood to different degrees, from being in an intense black mood to having a sense that things feel off. This is because female sex hormones regulate moods and how we experience pleasure, which is why many women notice they don't enjoy things as much anymore.

Feeling unmotivated is also common because motivation levels are linked to pleasure. Typically, we feel motivated because we experience pleasure as a reward for making an effort. Imagine you decide to cook your evening meal from scratch. You really enjoy it and feel pleased when you notice you're less bloated than usual and, as a result, have a better sleep. Your brain registers the positive experiences and links them to the effort you went to. The next night, you recall the benefits of cooking and are motivated to do it again.

Say you didn't enjoy the meal and had cravings soon after because you felt deprived. In that case, your brain associates a negative effect with cooking, and you won't be motivated to cook next time. This is what causes motivation to drop.

Living without experiencing life's little rewards and pleasures drags us down. We crave feeling good again, so we seek it elsewhere. Enter sugar, chocolate, prosecco and ultra-processed foods. We get an instant pleasure surge from the dopamine hit these foods give us, so it's no wonder we crave them.

Without motivation, we can't be bothered to do the extra work that switching to a healthier diet creates. With a low mood, the added discomfort of feeling hungry or going without your favourites is too much. One client told me she couldn't bear to go on a diet because she simply couldn't cope with feeling hungry. Life was simpler in our 20s and 30s, and our motivation levels were naturally higher. We could put up with the extra work and deprivation that comes with a new diet and exercise programme. Now we can't.

Overwhelm & brain fog

Feeling overwhelmed is an awful symptom, and I liken it to feeling like a rabbit trapped in headlights. You feel stunned at the prospect of everything you have to do, yet can't even make simple decisions. With brain fog, you can't think clearly. Going about your day in this state is exhausting and leaves you physically spent. If you've always been proud of your capacity to get stuff done, brain fog and overwhelm chip away at your self-worth and even your identity. Not being able to cope with home life and struggling to maintain your career is terrifying, adding even more stress to your life.

In relation to mealtimes, as daft as it sounds, you can't decide what to cook. I often stand in front of cupboards, trying to figure out what I feel like eating. On the bad days, I pick at things while trying to make up my mind and end up eating loads of rubbish and snacking all day because I've not eaten properly. Without the capacity to think logically about your options and link them back to your goals, you take the easiest and usually more unhealthy choice.

Other symptoms

There are many more symptoms of menopause, and each woman will experience a different combination. Some symptoms come and go, and others may be more consistent.

- Hair loss or thinning
- Muscle pain
- Painful sex
- Low energy

- Breast pain and tenderness
- Joint pain
- Abdominal pain
- Allergies
- Dizziness or feeling faint
- Heart palpitations
- Tingling hands & feet
- Frequent urination
- Difficulty concentrating and forgetfulness

Regularly experiencing these symptoms makes life harder. Layering them over everything else we've got on pushes us to the limit.

Getting professional help

If you feel like you are experiencing perimenopause or menopause symptoms, your first call should be your GP. Ideally, all GPs would be trained to spot perimenopause symptoms and offer women advice about their options to manage this. However, there is a variation in the standard of care you can expect from one practice to another. To get the most from your appointment, do some research first. One of the best places to start is with the Balance App. It was created by Dr Louise Newson, a GP and menopause specialist and an active campaigner for improving menopause services. It is a reliable and free source of up-to-date advice and even includes information to give your doctor if they aren't as clued up as you'd like them to be. HRT can help alleviate many symptoms; however, not all women can or indeed want to take HRT. Your doctor can advise you on all the options, which are also explained on the Balance App.

An Unhealthy Relationship with Food

When is the last time you felt truly hungry? We no longer eat because we need fuel. Instead, we eat to celebrate and relax, to alleviate boredom and make us feel better when we're lonely or unhappy. Giving people food shows we care, and we feel good when we treat our loved ones. We're even told by raising the metabolism, snacking helps us lose weight. The days of eating three square meals a day are long gone, and we've become a nation of constant grazers.

Whilst there's nothing wrong with the occasional indulgence, the truth is many of us overeat day-in-day-out. Rising obesity levels bear witness to this, with around 75% of people over 45 now either overweight or obese.[7]

Every time we eat, we top up our energy levels. One of the reasons we store body fat is to allow us to go for prolonged periods without eating. We can use body fat for energy when there's no food available. But by constantly eating, we never need to tap into our fat stores and add to them instead. It's like keeping your phone plugged in and never running down the battery.

Giving up snacks is not as easy as it sounds. We crave the high we get from hyper-palatable food and face constant temptation because we are surrounded by food wherever we go. Our natural hunger and appetite signals have been dulled, and we never feel full or satisfied. Cravings are powerful and difficult to ignore and ruin many diets. If cravings are one of your biggest weight-loss blockers, you must learn how to overcome them and understand why you eat when you don't feel remotely hungry.

We were all born with perfectly tuned hunger hormones that signal when we're hungry and full. This system governs our appetite, so we eat the right amount to maintain our ideal, natural weight. Sadly, many of us have lost this connection with our instincts and no longer recognise these signals.

I'm lucky to know someone whose hunger hormones are in perfect working order - my daughter. She will not eat unless she is hungry. Then, as soon as she's full, she puts down her fork and cannot stomach another mouthful. It doesn't matter if there's a tempting dessert on offer; she won't touch it. By unfortunate comparison, I never notice feeling full. I'll finish everything on my plate and happily carry on eating dessert, cheese, chocolate – whatever's on offer. Of course, I eventually stop, usually because there's nothing left or because I'm too embarrassed to carry on. While it's highly likely my daughter will stay naturally slim, I've had to learn to rein in my eating habits.

True hunger builds slowly. At first, hunger pangs come and go, gradually intensifying until they're persistent and hard to ignore. Blood sugar dips, and we feel irritable and shaky and have a strong desire to eat. Our mouth waters at the sight of food, which signals the digestion process is starting. The first bites we take are delicious because taste buds are at their most sensitive, and as we eat, their sensitivity diminishes. This means as we continue to eat, food tastes less appetising, and our attention shifts to the feeling of fullness. Eventually, our body senses we've eaten enough. To signal this, we stop enjoying what we're eating and put down our forks. That's precisely what happens to my daughter. Still, many people no longer experience this and cannot resist the constant urge to eat. Why can't we stop eating?

Survival instinct

From an evolutionary point of view, survival depended on our ability to seek out and consume food. Human brains are hard-wired to enjoy eating and be distracted by hunger until we satisfy our need for food, not knowing how long it will be until our next meal. We experience the same primal drive to eat today, except evolution hasn't caught up with the fact that most of us have constant access to thousands of calories.

Craving nutrition

What we eat influences how much we eat. On average, almost 60% of the total calories we eat in the UK come from ultra-processed foods.[8] These include everyday staples like white bread and bagels, chicken nuggets, oven chips, pizza, flavoured yoghurts, ready meals, crisps, carbonated drinks, fruit squash, sweets, chocolate, biscuits, and cakes.

Ultra-processed foods are mass-produced and generally made from cheap, unhealthy ingredients: sugar and syrups, refined flours, and refined vegetable oils. Unfortunately, the combination of high sugar and high fat in ultra-processed foods is delicious to eat. The pleasure we get from these foods is so intense that we're driven to keep eating them. Food companies are well aware of this phenomenon, and our constant desire for them drives sales. But the addictive taste isn't the only reason we keep eating them.

It's now thought we need specific amounts of protein and other nutrients. Despite being high calorie, many ultra-processed foods are low in protein and essential nutrients, meaning we're not getting enough nutrition. As a result, we keep eating, going way over our calorie requirements and wreaking havoc on our hunger hormones and blood sugar. This is why we can't stop eating.

Sugar crashes

Many convenient snack foods are high in sugar and refined carbohydrates. They might taste great and give us an immediate energy boost, but this is because they are quickly converted to glucose which spikes blood sugar. This is a problem because too much sugar in the blood is toxic, so a hormone called insulin is released to remove it. It has to go somewhere and can either be stored in the liver, the muscles or fat cells. But unless we do lots of vigorous exercise or have a demanding manual job, the liver and muscles can't absorb much. Instead, the excess is stored in fat cells, which is how too much sugar makes us fatter.

As blood sugar levels return to normal, some insulin remains which causes blood sugar levels to drop too far, triggering a sugar crash. This is why you feel ravenous a couple of hours after a high-carb breakfast and can't last until lunch.

Habitual eating

We love routines, rituals, and habits and most of us have a tendency to create habitual eating patterns which add hundreds of calories in addition to main meals. We crave something sweet after every meal and don't think twice about having popcorn at the cinema, crisps with beer, biscuits with tea, and hoovering up the kids' leftovers. Individually, these indulgences wouldn't be a big deal, but the reality is that they become regular occurrences.

Habits are actions we do without thinking, and it's the same with snacking habits. We tend overlook them, forgetting they each add more calories, yet hidden habits like these will undermine any diet you go on.

Eating for pleasure

Sometimes we just fancy something nice. Food is an easy source of pleasure, and we feel we deserve treats when we work so hard. Many women experience more sweet cravings around menopause. Sugary snacks give us instant energy and a hit of pleasure. If you're feeling down or tired, it's a guaranteed way to give yourself a much-needed boost.

Emotional eating

Many of us reach for something to eat when we're bored, lonely, sad, or anxious. Emotional eating is one of my main triggers, but only certain situations make me crave food. When I'm bored, I rummage through the cupboards. When I feel overwhelmed, I use eating as an excuse to take a break. If I feel anxious and restless when I'm stuck at home, my cravings go through the roof. Yet, if I have a row and feel upset, I can't eat at all.

Negative emotions create uncomfortable sensations in the body, and instead of dealing with them, we suppress them with food. We ignore these feelings for many reasons: conditioning, inconvenience, fear, and trauma. Eating pushes down the emotion and creates a temporary distraction. Emotional eating is usually a reaction to negative emotions, and it's no coincidence that we tend to crave highly processed junk foods that give us a high. They might temporarily lift our mood, but it doesn't last. Because it hasn't been acknowledged and processed, the emotion is still there, so the craving persists.

Food is sometimes used as a coping mechanism for people who have experienced abuse or trauma. In these circumstances, specialist help is needed, and sufferers need support to process their experiences. Others eat to avoid dealing with complex issues in their lives, like failing relationships or coming to terms with bereavement. In these cases, you may also benefit from professional support.

Sugar addiction

Many people say they're sugar addicts, but that's not usually the case.

Addictive eating is characterised by extreme out-of-control eating, and binges can last several days. To counter the inevitable weight gain, sufferers may use laxatives or make themselves vomit. This behaviour is classified as an eating disorder and needs professional help.

Whether it is possible to be addicted to specific foods is a hotly debated topic. It involves understanding how the brain responds to known addictive substances (like class A drugs) and whether foods can cause identical reactions.

Some people notice they find it difficult to moderate certain foods. They mostly have normal eating habits, but the floodgates open when they give in to weaknesses. For example, after eating a couple of squares of chocolate, they finish the whole bar. Or a couple of biscuits turns into an entire packet. It's easy to see how these episodes undo weight loss efforts; hundreds of calories can be eaten in a few minutes. In these instances, it's often easier to accept you need to give up trigger foods than try to eat them in moderation. If you can't let go of trigger foods, you may need help from a specialist.

Stuck in the kitchen

If you spend a lot of time in the kitchen, you're surrounded by temptation. We increasingly live and work in our kitchens, and when food is only an arm's reach away, it's hard to resist.

Low hunger hormones

A minority of people are thought to have naturally low levels of hunger hormones, preventing them from sensing they're full and making it hard to stop eating. But for most, it's more likely that the combination of societal influence, habits, and the food we eat that is responsible for losing the connection between eating and hunger.

True hunger

When you dramatically cut calories on a diet and eat portions that are too small, you get cravings because you are hungry. The body sends powerful signals to eat more if you don't eat enough. Many people find they don't have time to eat properly. Instead of eating regular, balanced meals, they graze throughout the day and end up starving and unable to wait any longer. One client asked for help breaking her junk food habit. She wanted to eat healthier meals but couldn't resist fast food. It turned out she was barely eating all day. She couldn't face breakfast and was too busy at work to stop for lunch. By evening she was so hungry she couldn't resist the quickest option.

I grew up around women who delicately picked at meagre portions on small plates while the men piled up big plates and ate with gusto. It's not uncommon for women to feel like they should only eat tiny portions, but not allowing yourself to eat appropriately sized meals will only make you hungry sooner, leading to a constant grazing pattern.

Case studies

Debbie was a bubbly client in her mid-40s who asked for my help with a meal plan to help her lose weight. I asked her to keep a food diary for a few days so I could get a feel for how she usually ate. Her eating plan revealed perfectly healthy meals and provided no clues as to why she was three stone overweight. The culprit was constant snacking when she was working from home, treats with the kids at the weekend and picking leftovers from their plates. She hadn't kept these things from me on purpose. She genuinely didn't realise the extent of these extras and how many calories they added. Instead, she assumed she was eating the wrong things at mealtimes. She looked disappointed when I told her I wouldn't be giving her a new diet plan. I explained she'd get better results if she put her effort into eating less between meals; that was where the actual work was needed.

Amyna had just turned 45. She was borderline diabetic, and her doctor wanted her to lose weight to prevent her from developing full-blown diabetes. Despite her best efforts, the scales weren't changing. She was doing well with her meals, doing two PT sessions a week, and building up her walking. I was at a loss as to what to suggest next, so I tried to see if any food habits were lurking that we had overlooked. Her face lit up with recognition as I asked her to think about what could be stalling her weight loss. She had a jar of nuts next to the microwave. Every time she used it, she helped herself to a handful, which was several times a day. 'I'd never even noticed I was doing it!' she remarked.

Pat ate when she was lonely. Her sons were in their mid-teens and spent most of their time in their rooms. She and her husband had grown apart over the years, and their lives were becoming increasingly separate. Their relationship was at a stage where they didn't do anything together other than organise the family routine. She often felt trapped in the kitchen, waiting for the boys to come home from school or venture out of their rooms. Food was her only comfort. Deep down, she worried about what would happen to her marriage when the boys left home. In this case, food was distracting Pat from a daunting problem. When you take away food from this situation, you confront the root cause, which in this case was her failing marriage. In these circumstances, professional support may be needed because overeating is a symptom of a different issue.

Hilary wanted to drop a couple of dress sizes for a holiday to celebrate her 50th birthday. When we did our first consultation, she admitted she had a big snacking habit and knew it was behind her weight gain. Reducing the temptation to snack meant eating filling, satisfying meals, and I recommended increasing the amount of protein for main meals and eating extra vegetables. Initially, this worked brilliantly, and she easily lost 4lb within a couple of weeks. However, after this, her weight loss stalled. By the fourth week, she'd put half the weight back on. Because she was doing so well, she thought she could relax her diet. She discovered some low-calorie alternatives to her favourite snacks and started eating fruit between meals. She thought this was OK because they were healthier snacks than before, but they still added enough calories to stall her weight loss.

Karen was a client who wanted to lose weight too. While she was happy to make changes, she wasn't prepared to give up her snacks at the end of the day. For her, the ritual of making herself a little platter of snacks and curling up on the sofa after finishing her chores signalled the moment she could finally relax. Fortunately, creating a healthier lifestyle doesn't mean giving up everything you love. You can choose what you want to keep eating and decide what you can live without. Karen offset her evening snacks by having a smaller dinner and replacing starchy carbs (pasta, rice, potatoes, and bread) with extra vegetables and salad. She also checked the calories of her favourite snacks, so she didn't go overboard. She found this change easy because it was a win-win; she could eat with the family and still enjoy her me-time later.

Sabotage

Sameera stepped on my scales. No change since last week. I pulled the tape measure around her waist, praying I would be able to give her good news about her measurements instead, but it wasn't going to be this week. She'd been coming to me for a few months to train twice a week. Her fitness and energy levels were improving, but she had barely lost any weight. Any time she did lose some, she put it straight back on the following week. Sameera was a borderline diabetic in her late forties and had been sternly told to lose weight by her doctor.

Everything she told me suggested she was doing the right things. So, why wasn't her weight changing? Eventually, she revealed that her husband was sabotaging her diet. She'd stopped buying biscuits, crisps, and other food she wanted to avoid because if they were in the house, she had no willpower around them. As her habits improved, her husband developed a new one of his own. To get around the problem of having no treats in the cupboards, he began to buy chocolates and crisps on his way home from work. He made a big show about them relaxing and sharing them while they watched TV after dinner, and Sameera felt too guilty to turn him down.

Katy, 54, was desperate to shed weight because her back gave her constant pain, but her husband and teenage sons refused to make any changes. They insisted on her buying crisps, chocolate and biscuits, but she couldn't resist eating them herself when she was alone during the day. Her family wouldn't compromise at mealtimes either. The only way she could eat what she wanted was to cook herself a separate meal, and the extra work quickly became too much. Having to eat differently from the rest of the family felt isolating and was a blatant reminder of their indifference to her plight. Feeling utterly unsupported by her family meant her motivation was at rock bottom.

Anne-Marie was 49 and worked part-time. She was classified as obese and suffered from plantar fasciitis. Her son had behavioural problems and was a fussy eater. Her husband worked long hours and came home shattered, so it mostly fell to Anne-Marie to care for their son. Coping with his behaviour was exhausting. He made a huge fuss if she gave him healthier meals or said no to eating sweets after dinner. Most nights, she was too tired to argue and ended up sharing sweets with him while they watched TV. This was a complete blocker for her weight loss, and it continued to creep up.

Aadhya was 44 and had a rare health condition managed by medication with unpleasant side effects. Her doctor said losing weight would improve the condition to the extent she could come off the drugs. This was a big motivator for her, but still, she repeatedly lost and put on the same few pounds. She was from a big family and was very close to her mum. On her days off, her mum loved to spend time with her making traditional snacks and treats. Family get-togethers were always in the diary and centred around food. She found the pressure of not joining in too uncomfortable and, as a result, couldn't lose enough weight to come off her medications and just had to put up with the side effects.

Family sabotage is a common occurrence and a complex issue to deal with. The saddest thing is that all these women needed to lose weight for their health and were trying hard. Yet, each week they faced another disappointment because their attempts to make progress were entirely undermined by the very people to whom they were closest. They were incredibly frustrated. These women cared for and loved their families so much that they were prepared to jeopardise their health to keep their families happy. In return for their concessions, they received the opposite, a complete disregard for the suffering they were experiencing.

Away from home, sabotage comes at you from all angles. Passing on a colleague's birthday cake, swapping chips for salad or staying off alcohol on a night out can be met with serious objection. Being called out by others is embarrassing and ruins your enjoyment of an occasion. Whilst it's true the odd night out or slice of cake won't ruin your diet, that's not the point. You should be the one who chooses when you indulge and what you eat when you do. When you're a victim of sabotage, other people make the decisions for you and expect you to eat to please them.

How sabotage affects your weight

Sabotage is a problem because it can occur frequently, and the extra calories forced on you can be high enough for weight loss to stall. As people-pleasers, we don't want to say no. We worry our restraint will affect other people's enjoyment of an occasion. Besides, when we say no, we feel obliged to offer an explanation, which we know will be met with objection. No wonder we suspend our diets to deflect attention rather than risk being forced into an awkward conversation. Being honest with friends, colleagues, and partners about our weight is uncomfortable. Our motives for dieting are judged while we feel vulnerable about revealing our fears and worries about our weight and health.

Advertiser's Dream

Most of us are entirely unaware of how heavily food marketing influences our eating habits. We are bombarded by thousands of advertising messages a day, with a significant proportion coming from fast food outlets, food delivery services, soft drinks, confectionery, and processed food manufacturers. We're exposed to many times more adverts for ultra-processed foods than for natural foods like fruit and vegetables, dairy products, meat, and fish. And that influence is increasingly reflected in our shopping trolleys which contain more than 50% ultra-processed items.[(9)]

My dad coined the phrase, 'Advertiser's dream'. As children, when we saw tempting adverts on TV, we'd try to persuade him to buy the products for us. He'd laugh, telling us how daft we were falling for the messages in the adverts. He knew what he was talking about. As the Northern Advertising Controller of The Daily Mirror, he'd spent his career selling advertising space. He understood how advertisers carefully targeted their dream customers to persuade us why we needed to buy their products.

I followed my dad into the industry and worked in advertising agencies for over 25 years, witnessing many of these tactics first-hand. In one meeting, the Marketing Director of a well-known UK food chain boasted about a trial to encourage new fathers to buy beer when they bought nappies.

Retailers constantly analyse customer data to find new ways of tempting us to spend more when we shop. In this trial, they discovered new mothers often sent their partners out to buy emergency nappies in the evening. Looking at how they could use this insight to increase sales, they came up with the idea of putting beer on the shelves next to nappies. Knowing new fathers would be tired and stressed by their new arrival, they expected beer to be too tempting to ignore. And it was.

In supermarkets, ultra-processed food accounts for over 80% of shelf space.(10) Shopper tracking technology and purchasing data give brands and retailers powerful insights into customer behaviour. Food manufacturers compete to display their ranges at prominent locations, and premium products and unmissable offers are placed right where we can't miss them. Food packaging is designed to jump out at us, using colours, images, and vague descriptions that influence our perception of a product's taste, health benefits and environmental credentials. Tempting deals and special offers make us think we're getting good deals. They exploit our fear of missing out, and we end up buying more food than we need. All these initiatives have a massive influence on what we eat.

We're not just targeted when we are in stores, either. Food retailers and processed food manufacturers spend hundreds of millions of pounds on advertising every year. They reach us when we're using social media, watching TV, in the cinema, travelling, reading, and listening to podcasts and the radio. Despite spending vast sums of money, the food industry makes enormous profits, which proves how well advertising works. It works because they know all about us. They know when we're hungry and tired and stuck for ideas. They know we use food as a pick-me-up or as a treat between meals, and they encourage it. They even target our children using a concept called pester power, so kids nag us to buy the brands they want. Without us noticing, we're constantly reminded to eat and drink. With techniques like these, we've gradually been persuaded to fill our cupboards with more and more ultra-processed foods.

When we're not shopping for food, we're still under attack. Sweets and chocolate are placed alongside tills for petrol, newspapers, lottery tickets, coffee, and even clothes. Is it any wonder our waistlines are rapidly expanding when we're bombarded like this?

We've all popped to the supermarket for one thing and left with bulging bags and a lighter wallet. How often do you have food in the fridge but order a takeaway instead? We all do exactly the same things, thanks to ruthlessly effective food marketing that constantly targets us and directly influences our behaviour.

How food marketing makes us fat

Being constantly surrounded by cheap, tempting treats and exposed to messages telling us to eat does affect our diets and, therefore, our waistlines. Our cupboards are filled with tasty snacks we can grab anytime, and we do. Restaurant and takeaway portions are bigger and contain many more calories than their homemade alternatives.

As our diets include more ultra-processed foods, taste buds become used to highly palatable foods. They are so delicious that we are driven to eat larger portions and crave them often, increasing our calorie intake further.

Many of these foods are low in protein and other essential nutrients but high in sugar, refined flour, and cheap oils. New research suggests we overeat these foods because our appetites are governed by how much nutrition is in our food. We pile our plates with too many calories and crave constant snacks because what we are eating is devoid of the nutrition our bodies desperately need.

• PART TWO •

A DIFFERENT APPROACH

The Power of Food and Exercise

It wasn't until I had a crush on a boy who was an amateur athlete that I took an interest in fitness at 15. First, I joined his ju-jitsu club, and then I bought a road bike so I could get there. We dated for a few months before he dumped me, but my love affair with exercise continued until I went to Uni. Then drinking, clubbing, and late-night takeaways took over.

By my mid-20s, my party lifestyle was showing, and I was a couple of stones heavier. When one of my boyfriend's friends told me I looked pregnant, I was mortified and decided to take up running. Running didn't come naturally. At school, I was always one of the last in races and was in awe of the lithe girls who could effortlessly sprint. There was a 100m stretch in the local park where my primary school sports days had taken place, and I decided that was as good a place to start as any. As I crossed the finishing line, my lungs were on fire, and I was gasping for breath, my body shocked by the unfamiliar exertion. For some reason, despite feeling on the verge of collapse, I kept it up, going three or four times a week. I couldn't run for long, so I alternated between walking and running, memorising the distance between trees and lampposts along the route, so I could push myself to run a bit further each time. I'd started running to lose weight, but it was a completely unexpected side effect that got me hooked.

My job demanded long hours, and, in the run-up to an important client meeting, I was sat alone in the office, tapping away at spreadsheets late into the evenings. Normally these lonely shifts were a slog, but this time I was in a great mood. I was in awe of how sharp my mind was and how I could concentrate intensly for hours. My body didn't look any different yet, but my energy was on another level, and I vowed to stick with the running.

In my late-30s, I began to experience terrible trouble staying awake at my desk after lunch. I still wince at the memory of losing the battle to stay awake in a small group presentation after going out for a team pizza. My usual lunches were sandwiches, and I can't remember why, but one day I decided to switch things up and had some nuts and a tub of cottage cheese. That same afternoon I didn't feel sleepy and powered through my work. I hated having to fight the urge to sleep at my desk, and when I realised what I ate could make such a difference, I stuck with it. Did I miss eating sandwiches? Maybe at first, but I soon got used to my new lunches and enjoyed them just as much. The benefits significantly outweighed the tiny sacrifice of not eating a couple of slices of bread.

We've become so used to eating ultra-processed foods that we don't notice how they affect us. I remember the first time I ate a McDonald's. My aunty worked for The Sun newspaper, and every day for a week, you had to cut out a little coupon from the paper and tape it to a printed form. When you had all 5 tokens, you got a free Big Mac. She collected the tokens from the papers in her office and gave my sisters and me the vouchers. It was so exciting to walk in and order without paying! But, straight after eating my much-anticipated burger, I had what felt like a brick in my stomach. It was as if the burger and bun had squashed up and stuck together to form a hard, uncomfortable lump.

My partner and I can tell when our kids have eaten certain takeaways; their eyes are puffed up the next day. The last time I had a Chinese, I felt like I had a raging hangover even though I hadn't had anything to drink. My face was so puffy I spent the day feeling excruciatingly self-conscious. It was so awful I've never had one since. If I'm ever tempted by the thought of one, I remember how I felt and wonder what on earth it did to my body, and decide it just isn't worth it.

Eating well isn't complicated, and the truth is there are no miracle diets. Unfortunately, cooking has become an optional chore because food manufacturers and fast-food outlets do most of the work. All we have to do is open a packet or an app. In the same way we'd never go back to washing clothes by hand, we're understandably reluctant to go back to peeling and chopping.

It's crucial you believe eating healthier and moving more will make you look and feel so much better. But it will take longer to notice a difference in how you look, compared to noticing how much better you feel.

Diet and exercise will improve your body shape, but the gradual changes make it hard to notice yourself. Your clothes might feel looser, but you'll be pushed to see significant changes by obsessively checking yourself in the mirror. If you're just relying on your reflection to motivate you, don't bother. Ultimately, how you feel will have a much more profound effect on your motivation than what you look like.

Nearly all my clients started exercising to lose weight but found the immediate energy boost made the biggest impact on their lives, and that's why they kept exercising. After switching to home-cooked meals, they felt less bloated, they could think clearer and had less brain fog, which also improved their mood. These benefits come surprisingly quickly. Stick with it for longer, and you'll be more resilient to stress, have better sleep and even clearer skin, as well as slowly starting to notice those extra pounds melting away.

Use the negative feelings you experience from eating unhealthy foods to increase your resolve to avoid them. You've probably created negative associations with some foods already. If a particular food made you ill in the past, it might have put you off for life. Vegans and vegetarians create such strong associations between meat and animal welfare that they don't need willpower to resist eating it. Many will openly admit to missing a bacon butty, but even if they were starving and hours away from being able to eat, they'd turn one down. I'm sure you've felt nauseous after eating a decadent dessert after a big meal. I certainly have. That's your body telling you that you've overloaded your stomach to the point where it's struggling to cope. Most people don't eat Foie Gras anymore because even meat eaters can't condone the idea of force-feeding a duck. If you want the willpower to pass on dessert when you're full, remind yourself that you're forcing food down past your natural limit.

As you make healthier changes to your lifestyle, do everything you can to create a positive association between diet and exercise and the benefits you experience. Constantly remind yourself that healthy food and exercise really do have the power to make you look and feel better. This can make a massive difference to your willpower.

Why It's Different for Women

My partner recently wanted to lose a few kilos. He decided to do an intermittent fasting diet for six weeks. He lost the weight he wanted and has since kept it off. That's it.

Infuriating, isn't it? Tim does a physical job and works incredibly hard. Whilst he was dieting, he ate breakfast and then worked all day without eating before having his tea. He counted calories for both meals to stay within the recommended calories and just got on with it. He never complained about being starving. I never found him rooting through kitchen cupboards trying to sneak a snack or tormenting himself with what he could fit into his calorie allowance. There was no drama or mental anguish. He made his meals, ate them, and then carried on with whatever else he was doing.

I've heard similar stories from other women about their husbands. One woman told me her husband had started working out. He had no problem leaving her and the kids to go for a run in the evening. If his workouts clashed with work, he simply told them he'd call back later. One weekend when she went away, leaving him with the kids, he arranged for a babysitter so that he didn't miss his session at the gym.

When we try to start a diet or exercise routine, we have such a different experience. We make ourselves so available to everyone all the time we find it impossible to leave them to it and would be too worried about what we'd come home to. And we definitely wouldn't feel comfortable expecting work to fit around our exercise schedule!

We're at a biological disadvantage from an eating point of view too. Behavioural studies have shown women are more likely than men to overeat when given tempting food or when they're feeling emotional. There's also scientific evidence that women have a harder time controlling their hunger than men and feel hungrier sooner after eating.[(11)(12)] Men are more able to override their brain's hunger signals, meaning they can resist their favourite foods while we can't. It's not fully understood why this is the case, but it's possibly linked to our sex hormones. Regardless of the cause, the bottom line is it's a fact we find it more difficult to give up our favourite foods when we diet, and we struggle when we go too long without eating.

So, if we want to lose weight, it seems we have to rewire our brain, override our hormones, give up our jobs and go and live on a desert island. As depressing as this might sound, the one thing I desperately want you to accept is that it's not your fault if you've struggled to stick with a diet and you are not lazy or greedy. So many factors conspire against us, and not one of them is down to your failings as an individual. I sincerely hope that makes you feel better.

Anyway, none of this means you can't lose weight or adopt a healthier lifestyle. All it means is we must take a different approach. Losing weight is different for women, and it changes again as we approach menopause. This is why we can't just jump straight into the topics of food and exercise.

Diet and exercise may be the things that govern weight loss, but we need to figure out how to stay focused and consistent because this determines whether or not we do the actual work to make it happen.

Building Motivation

Deep down many women sense they're not as motivated anymore, and it's true that hormonal changes make us feel like we can't be bothered. I used to have no problem avoiding foods that weren't good for me. I was clear about what I did and didn't want to eat and found it easy to turn down the things I knew I was better off not eating. But over the last few years, I noticed that I didn't care as much anymore. If I felt like I wanted cake, I ate it. The trouble was that I felt like cake more and more often, and my overall diet gradually worsened too, which took its toll on my weight, digestion, and mood. But it's not just our attitudes to food that can shift at this time of our lives.

I bumped into a friend recently who I hadn't seen for a couple of years. She'd worked throughout lockdown for the NHS without a break whilst doing holistic therapy in her spare time. As we caught up on each other's news, she explained she'd given up her main job and had barely worked for months. She said she just didn't have the motivation anymore but was absolutely fine with it and was actually enjoying doing so little. Her finances had taken a hit, but again she was OK that she had less money; having more time to take things easy was proving worth it.

Menopause is a time of change and transformation. Sometimes, we need to rest and recover or disrupt established routines so we can discover something new. If our body is screaming at us to do nothing, maybe we should listen.

But what happens when you decide you do want to change or aim for a new goal and can't be bothered to pursue it? We can't sit around waiting for motivation to arrive like a parcel we've ordered from Amazon; we must cultivate it instead.

Adopt a priority mindset

Think back to a time in your life when you really wanted something. A new career or house, a relationship, or to start a family. No one waved a magic wand to shower you with extra time, energy, or money to help you achieve your goal. But once you'd made up your mind, nothing could stop you from getting what you wanted. Of course, you had setbacks, and things didn't always go to plan, but you never lost sight of your goal and had to be creative and resourceful to make it happen.

We're constantly reprioritising things to fit everything into our day. The people who shout loudest get most of our attention, while the smallest voice – our own – fades into the background. We 'forget' to go to the gym or prepare a packed lunch, not because we can't be bothered, but because we're too busy reacting to everyone else. Until you become top of your list, others will always get the lion's share of your energy and attention.

True priorities are powerful. The way the world mobilised in response to the Covid-19 pandemic was staggering. Protecting the lives of the global population and reducing the risk of overwhelming health infrastructures were given unprecedented priority status. The scale of resources put into testing, vaccination research and rollout, and social interaction in healthcare, school, travel, and employment were astounding. Of course, there were failures, controversies, and inequalities, but the rate at which the world reacted is mind-blowing. None of these things could have possibly happened without Covid assuming such a top priority status.

Sleep has been one of my top priorities for years. I barely ever have to slog through the day shattered because I always sleep well. This is no happy accident; I've worked at it for years, and I rarely let anything get in the way of a good sleep. I go to bed and get up around the same time nearly every day, even on holiday, and I've trained myself to switch my brain off when I go to bed. A few years ago, we went through a particularly tough time financially. We missed a couple of mortgage payments and didn't know where our next pay check was coming from. Even then, I slept fine. I did plenty of worrying during the day but could switch my mind off at bedtime. Now, I don't have to think about sleep. I just do it because it's become a deeply ingrained habit. All I have to do is protect my routine by saying no to anything that might affect it.

What could be more important than your well-being? How important is staying fit and healthy for your future? Improving your health demands lifestyle changes, and the only way to make this happen is to prioritise it over everything else. Each day you must make conscious decisions to eat well and move and fiercely protect these vital things from interference by others. Get comfortable letting other people wait while you take care of your business first. Shifting your priorities doesn't mean other things won't get done; they just get done later.

There are times in my life when I clearly remember deciding to make something happen. When I got together with my current partner, I can still recall the exact moment I vowed I would do everything to make our relationship work. My resolve was decisive. I wasn't hoping things would work out; I was deciding they would. One of my lovely clients recently returned from visiting her mother, who lives abroad. She hadn't seen her during lockdown, and her mother had had a health scare, so this was a special holiday. After spending much longed-for time just sitting and chatting with her mum, she told me that while she'd been there, she'd had a lot of time to think and had decided things had to change and that this was her time. I had to hold back the tears and just gave her a big hug. This lady had an incredibly busy lifestyle, I was in awe of how she managed it, but it was taking its toll on her health and well-being. I'd asked her many times to focus more on herself, but she always had reasons she couldn't. We can't be nagged into things; we must decide for ourselves.

All you need to begin with is that lightbulb moment where you decide that now is your time. It doesn't matter if you have no idea how you'll manage it. It's like planting a seed. You put it in some soil, water it, and leave it in the sun. Nothing happens for a while, and then the first tiny shoots appear. Gradually, new leaves form, and eventually, it becomes a beautiful, healthy plant. All you have to do is nurture the idea of putting yourself first. As the idea settles, you'll instinctively come up with ways to make it happen. It might be something small at first, but then, encouraged by those first small steps, you'll get braver and figure out how to make further changes.

You don't need an elaborate plan to get started because we can always work things out along the way once we've set our minds to something. More than anything you have read so far, I want you to realise that nothing will change unless you commit to putting yourself first.

Goal Setting

Once you've committed to prioritising yourself, the next step is to decide on your goal. It's a fact that people who have clear, specific goals are more successful than those who don't. But first, you need to uncover what you truly want and why it is important to you.

Wanting to lose weight is an obvious goal. But sometimes, people fail because, deep down, they're not that bothered about it. They've just been telling themselves they should for years and have almost convinced themselves it's what they want. But when push comes to shove, they can't change their diet or establish a regular exercise routine because losing weight isn't truly important to them.

Often when we imagine ourselves losing weight, we conjure an image of a perfect body. I hate to crush your goals, but that doesn't exist. Why am I saying this when I've written a weight loss book? Being in a healthy weight range does improve your general health and risk of many common diseases, and that's a fact. But it doesn't guarantee you'll be happy or confident in your skin. If self-confidence is your goal, then you'll need more than a meal plan.

I was dumped by a boy when I was 13 because my legs were too fat. A gang of us had been swimming, and afterwards, this lad came right out and told me to my face that was the reason. He'd seen me in a swimsuit and didn't like what he saw. It's no coincidence that I went on my first diet when I was 13 and spent the next 36 years hating my legs. For most of that time, I was on and off diets, hoping to lose the fat and smooth the cellulite. Only in the last couple of years have I finally realised it's not going to happen and, instead, decided to make peace with them. Having thin legs is a pointless goal because, genetically, I can't change them. When I tried to diet to change my legs, it frustrated me and got me down. I'd make a huge effort, and when I looked in the mirror, I saw the same dimply legs and chunky knees looking back at me.

I've done plenty of soul-searching and have finally found a goal I believe in. I want to put two fingers up to growing old gracefully. I want to stay strong and mobile, so I can have great adventures when my teenager goes to university. That goal has real significance to me, and I've decided that it will happen rather than hope it will. That shift in priority really fires me up. I never forget about it, and it's always somewhere in my consciousness. When I'm tired or low, it's easy for me to latch onto my little dream and remind myself that five minutes of chopping some vegetables will make a difference. I keep exercising because I notice little aches and strains when I don't, and I'm committed to staying strong. I have a little mental picture of myself living my best life, which spurs me to keep going, even when I don't feel like it.

When you've found your true, motivating goal, proudly take ownership of it. Tell anyone who'll listen and make it as real as you can. Many women are embarrassed to say what they want, fearing judgement or being put down and told they're being unrealistic. People are happy for us to sit on the sidelines while we help them achieve their goals and feel threatened when they learn we have dreams and ambitions of our own.

Other's daren't admit to their deepest desires because they don't see how they can achieve them when they're so busy. So, they ignore it to avoid being disappointed. Suppressing what we want festers and eats away at us. It's time to stop caring what anyone else thinks. Giving yourself permission to unapologetically do what you want is incredibly liberating after years of holding back.

Goal setting exercise

This exercise will help you uncover your goal and clarify why it is so important to you.

Question	**Notes**
What is my goal?	
Why is this goal so important to me? *Dig deeper to uncover the driver behind your goal that is the most powerful motivator. To find this, ask yourself why 4 or 5 times until you find the driver that is most meaningful to you. For example, I want to drop a dress size for my holiday.*	Why #1 Why #2

<table>
<tr>
<td>Why #1
Because every time I go on holiday, I'm heavier than the previous year and feel so self-conscious and cross with myself

Why #2
Because I want to relax and enjoy my holidays instead of obsessing about how I look

Why #3
Because I've had enough of feeling bad about myself and eating for the wrong reasons

Why #4
Because it's stopping me from enjoying my life, not just my holidays

Why #5
Because my children will be leaving home in a few years and I want the confidence to build a new life for myself when they've left.</td>
<td>Why #3

Why #4

Why #5</td>
</tr>
<tr>
<td>Why is this goal so important to my future self?

Build as detailed a picture as possible to visualise how this goal will transform your future. The more detail you create, the more realistic this goal will become, which helps achieve it.</td>
<td></td>
</tr>
</table>

If I don't achieve my goal, how will it affect me? *Thinking about the consequences of not achieving your goal will provide additional motivation to act.*	
If I don't achieve my goal, how will I feel? *Imagining the emotional consequences of failing adds more power and motivation to succeed.*	
What do I have to do to achieve my goal? Be as specific about the actions you must do to achieve your goal: What blockers do I have to address? What changes do I have to make to my diet, exercise, sleep, and stress levels? What actions can I realistically take right now in my life as it is?	
How will I feel when I've achieved my goal? *Describe this in as much detail as possible and try to bring it to life. Clearly visualising your goals is linked to a greater likelihood of achieving them.*	

When you have uncovered your goal, you will notice a renewed sense of motivation to get going. Keep your notes safe and revisit them frequently as a reminder of what you want and to help you push through when things feel hard.

Staying Connected to Your Goal

In 1961 a 200lb housewife called Jean Nidetch invited six overweight friends to her house. Jean had struggled with her weight since being a child. As an adult, she found her way to an obesity clinic in New York, where she lived and was given a strict diet. She still couldn't commit to the plan and made little progress. Frustrated by feeling that the women who ran the programme didn't understand her struggle, she abandoned the clinic and took matters into her own hands. She set up a small group of women who could meet and share their experiences and motivate each other. She eventually lost 70 pounds and went on to launch Weight Watchers.

Jean instinctively knew she needed more than a diet sheet. She needed to be accountable to others who knew exactly what it felt like to fight a losing battle with overeating. Connecting with like-minded women was key to finally overcoming her demons.

Weight Watchers still runs weekly meetings all over the world, which is proof of the difference that connection makes. Finding a weekly support group might be just what you need, or you can take the concept further and connect with your goal every day. This is how I managed to give up drinking alcohol three years ago. Most nights, drinking a glass or two of wine had become my routine. The day's worries evaporated the minute I settled onto the sofa, glass of wine in hand. I needed that moment. I was wrought with the stress of running a fledgling business, and the only time I could switch my brain off was when the wine came out, and the TV went on. I never felt drunk or had much of a hangover and reasoned that everything was fine and that most people did exactly the same.

I always enjoyed a January health kick after making the most of Christmas festivities, so decided to do dry January. I lasted three weeks before I gave in. I'd been in a foul mood the whole time, simply because I couldn't drink. Although it took me another six months to finally give up, that was when I started to realise my drinking was a problem.

Giving up drinking is not easy. We live in a society with a lot of pressure and expectation to drink, and I knew I needed support to manage such a significant change. Connection was how I did it. I joined an online support group, and first thing each morning, I read a few posts from other members. Reading their stories inspired me and fired my determination to stop drinking. Instead of lurking in the wings, I got involved, liking and commenting on others' posts. Then, I wrote a simple post setting my intention for the day and often received messages of encouragement from others. I kept this up for a few months until I felt I didn't need it anymore and had established a non-drinking lifestyle that I could confidently maintain. As I write this, it's been three years since I had a drink.

Connection was critical to my success because every day, it reinforced the pleasure of achieving small wins and kept me away from ruminating on the daunting prospect of never drinking again. It meant I started each day with a little celebration of how great it felt each morning to know I'd not drunk the night before. That simple victory spurred me on to keep going.

When temptation reared its head, instead of going into negotiations with that little voice that tries to convince you that one drink will be OK, I'd shift my thoughts towards how good I'd feel the following day. My attention was focused on achieving the wins instead of languishing in the pain of the struggle.

There are many parallels between giving up alcohol and cutting down on unhealthy, processed foods. But, unlike alcohol, we can't simply give up eating. We're surrounded by temptation wherever we are, and resisting our mental chatter is exhausting. Brains are experts at exploiting our weaknesses and persuading us to cheat on our diets. Instead of allowing your internal dialogue to torment you, Connection gives you something positive to focus on; that wonderful moment when you can say, I did it. I managed another day!

Connection works because it encourages us to tackle one day at a time. Any time we feel overwhelmed, we can just think about today. Our overactive brains will torment us with questions like, 'How will I manage this weekend/what will I eat at the party/can I eat desserts on holiday/can I ever eat chocolate again?' If we let this thinking run away with us, we quickly overcomplicate things. There's no need to think about the future or have every conceivable future scenario mapped out. Just do your best today.

Connection also has a significant role to play in long-term success. Research into the success of Alcoholics Anonymous found that support from a group strengthens confidence in being able to maintain new habits in situations where it's tempting to abandon them. With each small win, your confidence and motivation increase. Connecting with people who share the same challenges as you, is a game changer. We tend to imagine we are the only ones struggling. Realising what you are experiencing is very common, and not down to your personal failings, brings great relief.

Consistency is built up one meal and one day at a time until new lifestyle habits become automatic. It's said new habits take 21 days to create, but it can take significantly longer. You risk slipping back to your more familiar and comfortable behaviours until your new habits become ingrained. Spending a couple of minutes a day connecting to your goals and setting your intentions puts you in control of your day. It helps turn one great day into a long, consistent streak. And that's when you start to see results.

Making significant changes on your own can be daunting, so I'd like to invite you to join my free Facebook community so we can carry on this journey together.

Visit my website and find the link to join there:
www.gabrielleohare.com/book-resources

• PART THREE •

THE WEIGHT CHANGERS

By this point, you've accepted that the right food and exercise makes a difference to how you feel and are worth the effort. You've realised it's essential to become your number one priority. You've set yourself a goal you truly believe in and have decided on a way to connect with that goal every day. Now we can look at the specifics of what you have to do to lose weight and gain energy.

Diet & Nutrition

When it comes to losing weight, what you eat matters most. Exercising won't make up for cutting corners with your diet, so eating well must be your main priority. There is no magic formula; I haven't discovered anything new. Everything you'll read now is based on well-established nutritional science.

The formula for weight loss is simple and based on the following rules:

- Eat fewer calories than you need, but don't go too low
- Eat more natural, unprocessed foods and fewer highly processed foods
- Prioritise protein and vegetables and eat fewer carbs
- Make main meals satisfying, filling and enjoyable
- Try and leave 4 or 5 hours between meals
- Reduce snacking when not hungry and work to eliminate snacking triggers

The truth about calories

If you constantly eat more calories than you need, you will gain weight regardless of how healthy your food is. Knowing precisely how many calories you eat is difficult unless you count them. However, counting calories is a tedious chore for many women, including myself. Whether or not you want to count calories is up to you. I'll give you options to either count them or take a more intuitive approach, and you can decide which method suits you best.

Weight loss without counting calories

It is possible to lose weight without counting calories, but there may be some trial and error before you start to lose weight. To be sure you are losing weight, you will need to measure yourself weekly. Choose from measuring your chest, waist, and hips at the widest point, weighing yourself, taking progress photos or trying on the same item of clothing. Some people find weighing themselves triggering; others just see it as a number. I prefer to go on how my clothes feel. Just do what feels right to you.

To begin with, start with steps 1 to 3. If, after a few weeks, you aren't losing weight, add steps 4 & 5.

Step 1

Eat more natural, minimally processed and homemade foods. Natural food is more nutritious, and when we base our diet on it, we feel less hungry, and cravings disappear. Main meals should be appropriately balanced with the correct proportions of protein, carbohydrates and fat. Don't worry – it's not as complicated as it sounds, and I will explain more about how to eat later. There is also a recipe section at the end of the book and guidance for creating your own recipes.

Step 2

Leave 4 to 5 hours between meals. This gives us time to digest food properly and let our digestive system rest before we eat again. If you make main meals filling and well balanced, this shouldn't be too difficult. By the time your next meal comes around, you should be ready to eat but not starving.

Step 3

Reduce or eliminate snacks. Snacks are often the worst culprit for adding unnecessary calories and they quickly add up, even though we imagine we're not eating much. If you really can't wait until your next meal, choose snacks that include protein and carbohydrates. Stay mindful that too many low-calorie snacks still add up. Check the recipe section for ideas.

Step 4

Check Portion Sizes. If you're still not losing weight after a couple of weeks, the next step is to tweak portion sizes. Reduce the amount of fat and oils you add to meals and halve your usual serving size of bread, rice, pasta, potatoes and fruit. Don't skimp on the protein or vegetables, as they help fill you.

Step 5

Start paying attention to your hunger signals. Only eat when you're hungry and stop when you feel full.

If you follow these steps, you should lose weight without counting calories. However, if you still haven't lost weight and didn't cheat, I recommend counting calories for a few weeks. This gives you a more accurate picture of how much you're eating versus how much you should be eating.

Counting calories

Counting calories is more accurate, so you should see results sooner. By eating fewer calories than we need, the body burns fat to compensate for the deficit, which is how we lose weight. One pound of fat equals around 3,500 calories, so in theory, when we eat 3,500 calories fewer than we need, we lose one pound of body fat. To lose 1lb a week, you need to eat 500 fewer calories than you need each day.

It's tempting to go lower than this to speed things up; however, going too low will leave you feeling hungry and more likely to give up. If you're not losing weight, gradually reduce calories by 100 every couple of weeks until you start losing weight steadily.

Step One

Work out how many calories you need to eat for your age, size and current activity levels. You can do this easily using free online calorie calculators.

Step Two

Track the calories of everything you eat and drink. The best way to do this is with calorie-tracking apps, and MyFitnessPal is a good free one.

Apart from that, you should follow the same rules as above.

1. Eat more natural, minimally processed and homemade food

2. Leave 4-5 hours between meals and reduce snacking
3. Eat when you are hungry and stop when you are full

Setting Your Daily Calorie Target

The first step is to determine how many calories you should eat daily. The easiest way to do this is with an online calorie calculator.

Search Google or try this one:
https://www.omnicalculator.com/health/bmr-harris-benedict-equation

You'll be asked to input your height, weight, sex, age and how active you are. When you put in your data, you get the following results:

Your BMR. This is your Basic Metabolic Rate, the minimum number of calories you need to keep your body functioning, for example, if you spent all day in bed.

Your Total Daily Energy Expenditure (or TDEE) is the number of calories you need to maintain your current weight and carry out your usual activities.

Subtract 500 calories from the TDEE, and this is your daily calorie target.

For example, if your TDEE figure is 2,250 calories per day, subtracting 500 calories from this target gives you 1,750. This is how many calories to eat each day to lose weight.

Your daily calorie requirements will change as you become lighter and activity levels change. So re-check your calorie targets every month or two.

If all this sounds too much and you'd prefer to keep it simple, start by eating 1700 calories a week. If that doesn't result in a weight loss after a couple of weeks, drop it down by 100 calories every two weeks until you start to lose weight. Don't be tempted to go too low. The most sustainable option is to find the highest number of calories you can eat while still losing weight.

Tracking your Calories

To ensure you don't exceed your daily calorie target, track what you're eating. The easiest way to do this is to download an app.

Try MyFitnessPal, which is free. https://www.myfitnesspal.com/

It includes recipes, motivational success stories, nutrition advice and a large community you can join. There is plenty of advice on how to use the app to get the best results.

Tracking your Protein

As well as tracking calories, MyFitnessPal calculates how much protein, carbohydrate and fat you eat. Eating meals higher in protein helps regulate your appetite and minimise muscle loss. Aim for approx.imately 1g per Kg body weight, so if you weigh 70kg, you should aim for 70g of protein daily.

What you eat matters

Eating fewer calories than usual can leave you feeling hungry. The hungrier and more deprived you feel, the harder it is to stick to a diet. For the best weight loss results, count calories *and* choose nutritious, well-balanced food. If you count calories but disregard nutrition, you will feel hungrier, have more cravings, and find it harder to stick to your calorie limit.

What we eat affects how hungry we feel and whether we experience cravings. This is why it's essential to understand how food affects hunger, cravings, how much we eat, and even how many calories we absorb.

Give your body what it needs

We're happy to spend small fortunes on miracle face creams but forget nutritious food is more effective at slowing down the ageing process. Our bodies continuously rebuild themselves. Skin is completely renewed in 28 - 42 days, slowing to around 84 days after 50. Hair, nails, organs and the digestive system are constantly regenerating. Skeletons are entirely replaced every 10 years. Muscles are repaired and rebuilt when we exercise.

Natural, unprocessed food is the best source of raw materials for this constant regeneration. If you want to look your best and feel amazing for as long as possible, give your body the nutrition it needs to do its job correctly.

Avoid ultra-processed foods

Ready meals and takeaways might save us time and keep the kids happy, but we are short-changed on nutrition when we eat them. Evidence suggests getting most of your calories from ultra-processed foods increases how much people eat and leads to weight gain.[13] There's a lot of confusion about what ultra-processed food means and how to identify them.

Natural, unprocessed foods

These are foods that have had nothing done to alter their natural state. They include all fruit and vegetables, fish and seafood, poultry and meat, unsalted nuts and seeds.

Minimally processed foods

Still good for us, these foods have undergone some degree of natural or mechanical processing and may have small amounts of added salt and sugar. For example, butter and olive oil, tofu, fermented dairy, cheese, natural yoghurt, kefir, smoked salmon, frozen and canned fruit, vegetables and fish, canned and dried pulses, oats and rice.

Ultra-processed foods

Foods in this category are factory-made, using cheap ingredients. They mimic the appearance and taste of natural foods but are high in added sugars, refined flours, and refined vegetable oils. They rely on artificial additives to enhance flavour and texture. Their natural vitamins and minerals are often stripped out during production and replaced with synthetic versions. Stabilisers, dyes, and other bizarre-sounding ingredients are added to increase shelf life and make them hyper-palatable.

Foods from this category include white bread, bagels and wraps, flavoured yoghurts, pies, pastries, biscuits, pasta sauces, ice cream, crisps, confectionery, margarine, pizza, chicken nuggets, and ready meals. To check if something is ultra-processed, read the label on the packaging. If there are more than 5 ingredients, it's likely to fall into this category.

Vegans and vegetarians are increasingly targeted by food manufacturers keen to benefit from the growing trend in plant-based food. However, many plant-based foods are also classified as ultra-processed, so be wary when shopping. Check labels and choose natural vegan ingredients like nuts, seeds, pulses, vegetables, olive oil, coconut milk, tofu and wholegrains like oats, buckwheat and brown rice.

It's not only the lack of nutrition that's a problem when we eat ultra-processed foods. They are also known to have an insidious effect on our appetites:

- We overeat ultra-processed foods because they don't have enough nutrition. We need more nutrients than they contain, so we keep going in an attempt to meet our body's requirements, eating too many calories in the process.
- When we eat natural, unprocessed foods, some of the vitamins and minerals they contain are used for digestion. Because ultra-processed foods don't contain enough, we must use up our nutrient reserves to digest them. Startlingly, this means we can end up with fewer nutrients in our body after eating a highly processed meal.
- Processed foods are carefully designed to taste incredible, so we eat larger portions and buy them more often because we crave them.
- Many ultra-processed foods are high in carbohydrates and cause rapid glucose spikes in our blood. When we eat more than we can store in the muscles and liver, the excess is stored as fat.

We've become so used to eating processed foods we don't notice how bad they make us feel. One of my clients switched to mostly home cooked food. After a few weeks, she ordered a takeaway as a treat for her and her husband. The following day they were shocked by how rough they felt and how sluggish they were, and it lasted all day. Until this experience, they hadn't realised how much of a difference their new way of eating was making. Not only were they losing weight (without calorie counting), they were feeling more energetic and alert during the day.

This woman had a particularly stressful job and two young children, so making homemade dinners was a big ask. She soon noticed she was feeling more alert and energetic. She could manage her workload better and found it easier to cope with boisterous children in the evenings because she wasn't so tired and irritable. The benefits were so profound the extra cooking became worth it. Of course, they would still go out and have the occasional takeaway, but they knew they wouldn't return to their old habits.

Avoid sugar

On average, we eat 100g of sugar a day, and some people eat way more than this. When you understand how damaging sugar is, it can motivate you to ditch unhealthy, processed carbs and high-sugar snacks.

To give some context, a healthy individual will wake up with around a teaspoon of glucose (sugar) in their blood, around 5g. Constantly eating foods containing sugar and refined carbohydrates puts the body under stress because sugar is highly toxic and causes a host of problems[14][15][16] besides increasing body fat:

- Weight gain and obesity
- Tiredness and low energy
- Bloating

- Tooth decay
- Diabetes
- Cardiovascular disease
- High blood pressure
- Cancer
- Depression
- Worse joint pain and increased risk of developing rheumatoid arthritis
- Skin aging, damaging collagen and elastin to cause lines and sagging skin

Remember that refined carbohydrates behave in a similar way to sugar. This includes foods like white bread, bagels, pasta, rice cakes, crackers, oven chips, frozen pizza, cakes, pies, biscuits, pastries, confectionary, fruit juice and carbonated drinks.

Limit alcohol

The million-dollar question is can you drink and lose weight? Not only is alcohol high in calories, but it also makes people overeat and choose higher-calorie food than usual. A night of drinking and eating could easily add over a thousand calories. Alcohol is toxic and affects sleep quality and digestion. This is why you feel hungover the next day and crave comfort food.

Alcohol companies have been running multi-million-pound advertising campaigns for decades. And we've been conditioned to think drinking is glamorous and a prerequisite for a good time. But that's not true; we can enjoy socialising just as much without alcohol and waking up without a hangover after a great night out is a fabulous feeling.

Pubs and restaurants have an increasing choice of alcohol-free options, making it easier than ever to enjoy a night out without having to drink children's drinks. Steer clear of sugar-laden soft drinks and opt for alcohol-free beers, wines and spirits, which have the added bonus of being lower in calories than their alcoholic equivalents.

The bottom line is the more alcohol you drink, the harder it will be to lose weight. Most of us fool ourselves when we say we'll only have a couple. Alcohol weakens your resolve, so accept you'll get better results if you give up alcohol for a while.

What To Eat

The more you base your diet on natural, unprocessed foods, the better you feel and the easier you'll find it to lose and maintain weight. You get more protein, vitamins, minerals, and gut-friendly fibre from natural and minimally processed foods. You'll naturally eat fewer calories, experience fewer cravings, feel fuller for longer, and your energy will stabilise. We also absorb fewer calories from natural foods because digesting them is more complex. Depending on what you eat, as many as 10-25% of calories could be used during digestion.

Prioritise protein

Protein is a powerful macronutrient that we often don't get enough of. Hair, skin and nails need a good supply to keep them strong and healthy. It makes the collagen and elastin that keep skin smooth and firm, and muscles need it to repair and grow after exercise. Every cell in the body needs protein because it's essential for cell renewal and repair.

The older we get, the more essential it becomes, and it's especially significant for post-menopausal women. Research shows eating more protein improves body composition. Most of us would like our bodies to be more toned, and a higher protein diet can give you that.

In one study[17], researchers compared a group of post-menopausal women eating a low-protein diet with a group eating a high-protein diet. The women who ate the high-protein diet had less fat and more muscle, even though they ate more calories. They performed better at physical tests to measure their strength and fitness and reported fewer falls than the low protein group.

Eating more protein is a dieter's secret weapon. Cutting calories makes us hungry, and we can't ignore hunger long before giving in. Protein keeps us fuller for longer and reduces cravings, so it's easier to resist snacking. Aim to eat 1g of protein per kg bodyweight. So, if you weigh 70kg, aim for 70g. If you don't usually eat much protein, you might find this challenging at first. Gradually increase how much you eat until you get used to eating the proper amount. This is usually easy for meat-eaters but harder for vegetarians and vegans because the primary vegan sources: tofu, grains, pulses and nuts, are naturally lower in protein.

Sources of protein

Protein is made up of 21 different amino acids, and 9 are known as essential amino acids. These are especially important because we only get them from the food we eat. The other 12 can be synthesised in the body. Proteins which contain all 9 essential amino acids are known as complete proteins and include meat, fish, eggs and dairy. So, when you eat any of these, you get the 9 essential proteins together.

Many vegetarian and vegan proteins are incomplete and don't include all 9 essential amino acids. To get around this, eat several protein sources together; for example, combine lentils and rice, chickpeas and almonds.

Complete proteins

Red Meat
Poultry
Fish and Shellfish
Eggs
Natural Yoghurt – look out for Greek yoghurt and high protein brands with 6 -10g of protein per 100g
Cheese
Milk

Complete proteins vegan/vegetarian

Buckwheat – grains or flour
Tofu & tempeh
Quinoa
Hemp seeds
Chia seeds
Spirulina

Incomplete proteins vegan/vegetarian

Pulses & Legumes, e.g., chickpeas, kidney beans, lentils, peas, broad beans
Nuts and seeds, e.g., almonds, cashews, brazil nuts, walnuts, sunflower seeds, pumpkin seeds
Whole grains and oats

Make friends with fat

Fat tends to get a bad rap, but eating some is crucial as it contains essential fat-soluble vitamins, Vitamin A, D, E and K.

You may have heard about the Mediterranean Diet, considered one of the healthiest ways of eating. This diet is based on eating a wide variety of unprocessed foods, with lots of vegetables, fruits, whole grains and moderate amounts of meat, fish and dairy. It also includes plenty of healthy fats from olives, olive oil, oily fish, nuts, and seeds. People who eat a Mediterranean-type diet may live longer and be less likely to put on weight.

Fat is your friend if you want to enjoy food. We quickly get fed up with bland, boring food, and menopause can dull pleasure sensations from food. To make a healthy diet sustainable long-term, we need to eat food that rewards our senses in as many ways as possible. Fat adds flavour and richness to dishes and enhances the consistency and mouthfeel. We don't feel deprived when we enjoy what we eat, which makes us less likely to experience cravings later. Fat is also very filling and naturally reduces how much we want to eat.

Not all fats are equal. Avoid unhealthy fats in foods like pies, pastries, sausages, ready meals, margarine, vegetable and seed oils, shop-bought cakes, biscuits, pastries and bread, ice cream, fast food, crisps and frozen foods which have been deep-fried. Choose lean cuts of meat and remove excess fat.

Fat is still higher in calories than other foods, but a little can go a long way to make meals more enjoyable.

Healthy ways to add fat:

- Eat oily fish, such as mackerel, fresh or tinned salmon, sardines and anchovies two times a week
- Make dressings from extra virgin olive oil and add to salad or vegetables
- Add nuts, seeds, avocado and olives to salads
- Add a little butter to steamed and boiled vegetables
- Add coconut milk to curries for a rich, satisfying taste
- Choose full-fat dairy instead of low fat and eat smaller portions
- Add small amounts of cheese to salads, omelettes, and other recipes to add taste and texture
- Eat berries with a little single cream or Greek yoghurt for a low-carb sweet treat
- Enjoy a couple of squares of 70% dark chocolate
- Add a small handful of nuts or seeds to natural yoghurt

Be choosy about carbs

Carbohydrates are the most controversial of all foods. So, do carbs make you fat? Some do, and some don't. The carbs to watch out for are known as empty carbs. These include sugar, flour, breakfast cereals, noodles, rice cakes, cakes, biscuits, bagels, tortillas, garlic bread, frozen chips, crisps, pastries, ice-cream, desserts, sweets, flavoured and sweetened yoghurts, fruit juice, commercial smoothies, carbonated drinks. They are called empty carbs because their nutrients have been stripped out by processing, and as you have probably spotted, most are also classified as ultra-processed foods.

You're probably imagining the pleasure draining from your life because these are foods we love to eat. But we also find them hard to moderate and eating too many does affect your waistline. When we eat more carbs than our body can handle, they are stored as fat. Sugar highs are followed by crashes triggering intense cravings, making us eat more calories. The bottom line is that it's sensible to eat fewer empty carbs.

Pasta, bread, potatoes, and rice have a similar effect, but if you love eating them, you don't necessarily have to give them up. Simply have smaller portions of your favourites and eat them alongside decent portions of protein and vegetables. This way, meals are better balanced, so you stay full for longer, have fewer cravings and have stable energy.

Eat unlimited vegetables

All vegetables are carbohydrates and are full of vitamins, minerals and fibre. Increasing the variety of vegetables we eat improves gut health, which benefits digestion and immunity, so aim to eat a rainbow of vegetables each week.

Carbohydrate levels in vegetables vary. Green leafy vegetables such as cabbage, kale, spinach, lettuce and green herbs like parsley and coriander have the least. Other low-carb vegetables include cauliflower, broccoli, sprouts, peppers, cucumber, tomato, aubergine, squash, courgette, mushrooms, leeks, onions and garlic. Pile up your plate to combine tastes and textures and make meals interesting and filling.

Higher carbohydrate vegetables include root vegetables like carrots, parsnips, potatoes and sweet potatoes. Beans, peas and lentils are higher in carbohydrates and also contain protein in reasonable amounts, making them vegetarian and vegan staples. These are higher in calories than above-ground veg but are healthy and filling additions to meals.

Go easy on fruit

Fruit contains vitamins, minerals and fibre, but is also high in sugar, so don't eat too much. Snacking on fruit between meals isn't a good idea because it affects blood sugar in the same way as other sugary foods. Blueberries, raspberries and strawberries are good low-sugar options and make a filling breakfast when combined with pancakes or Greek yoghurt and nuts.

Make meals tasty & satisfying

It's vital that you enjoy what you eat if you want to change your diet for good. When we eat bland, dull food, we feel deprived because we've missed out on the pleasure of eating, which triggers cravings. If you don't enjoy your food, takeaways, snacks and convenience foods will quickly find their way back.

Don't let this happen! No one likes being plagued by cravings and the guilt that follows when you give in. You deserve to eat fabulous food that leaves you feeling satisfied and able to get on with the rest of your day without being preoccupied with eating something else. One client did fine in the summer but struggled when the weather got colder. She was happy eating salads when it was warm but needed something more comforting when it was chilly. Hearty soups and casseroles are still great options, so experiment until you discover new favourites that you can stick with long-term.

Leave 4 or 5 hours between meals

Our bodies are in either fat-burning mode or fat-storage mode. Every time we consume calories, we go into fat-storage mode. We only switch into a fat-burning mode when we've not eaten for several hours. But by eating constantly, we never give our bodies the chance.

Encourage your body to burn excess fat by going without food and calorific drinks between meals. As well as cutting out snacks, stick to water, black coffee and tea, and herbal teas. If this is a significant change, you need to be prepared. Decide in advance what time your meals will be. Make sure you have a hearty breakfast, so you don't get too hungry too soon. Having a set time to aim for gives you a better incentive to wait.

It's essential to make sure your meals are substantial and filling enough. If you skimp on portions, you won't last long without snacking. If you're used to eating little and often, you may worry that if your meals are too big you won't lose weight. It may take some trial and error to find the right sized portions that work for you.

Going without food for 4 to 5 hours may feel uncomfortable at first, because the body's fat-burning machinery is used to the constant supply of sugar. However, if you stick with it, you'll quickly adapt. Even if you have bigger meals than usual, it will still help you lose weight because you'll eat fewer calories overall by not snacking. You become more efficient at burning fat and spend more time burning it throughout the day.

Learn to manage cravings

Cravings have ruined many a diet, and most of us experience them. After going without sugar and processed foods, the brain starts to miss them and puts up a fight in the form of cravings. They will inevitably come up, so be prepared.

Surf the craving. Step away from food when a craving strikes and take a few steady breaths. Shift your attention away from the urge to eat and pay attention to any physical sensations you are experiencing. Is your mouth watering or your chest tingling? Does your throat feel tight? How is your breathing? Simply notice what's going on. Don't question it or judge yourself. As you pay attention to the sensations in your body, the craving will eventually disappear.

Distraction techniques. When you experience a craving, do something else to distract yourself. Clean your teeth. Call a friend. Go for a walk or take a bath. Anything will do. After a few minutes, you'll notice the craving has gone.

Look for the trigger. When you notice a craving, pay attention to what's going on to see if you can identify the trigger. Cravings are often a subconscious distraction technique to shield ourselves from things we find uncomfortable. When you find the cause, ask yourself what you really need right now. If you noticed the trigger was feeling restless, maybe you need to go for a walk instead. Take a walk, and the craving will go. This practice helps you spot and address patterns.

Indulge mindfully. Sometimes you might decide to indulge your craving. When you do, choose a modest portion and eat it slowly and mindfully. Really pay attention to it and savour every bite, so your brain registers the pleasure. Notice how you feel as you eat it and stop when you're no longer enjoying it.

Sample menu ideas

Breakfast	Blueberries, high-protein Greek yoghurt and a handful of nuts
Lunch	3-egg omelette with large mixed salad, dressed with olive oil and vinegar
Dinner	Beef Burger, Sweet Potato Fries, Homemade coleslaw

Breakfast	Pancakes with strawberries and raspberries
Lunch	Chicken and leek soup with grated cheese
Dinner	Prawn curry, with raita and poppadoms

Breakfast	Vegan Protein Smoothie
Lunch	Hummus with raw veg and small pitta bread
Dinner	Chickpea and lentil chilli with rice

Choose your food consciously

By now, I hope you have a better understanding of food and nutrition. Remember that some food is better for us than others and what we eat has a powerful effect on appetite and cravings. The more we eat natural foods, the easier it will be to maintain a healthy weight. Keep this front of mind to strengthen the link between food and health. If you consciously choose to eat ultra-processed foods now and again, that's OK. Use the 80:20 rule and be selective about what you want to eat, to find the balance that works for you.

My recipes & your recipes

You'll find a selection of quick and easy recipes based on what I cook at home at the back of the book. I've also included some helpful hints to help you create your own recipes.

Exercise

The truth about exercise and weight loss

More exercise isn't necessarily better when you are trying to lose weight. This is fantastic news if you thought you had to exercise for hours. Focusing on what you eat is more important because exercise burns far fewer calories than we imagine.

But when we diet, between 20% to 35%[(18)] of the weight loss comes from muscle, not fat. Imagine losing 10lb; as much as 3.5lb would be muscle. But this isn't the only way we lose it. Muscle mass naturally decreases with age, but during the five years after menopause, we lose it faster than at any other time in our lives. Allowing a diet to accelerate this is a terrible idea.

Fortunately, you can prevent this from happening by strength training while you diet. This is proven to be the most effective way to build muscle compared to other exercise types. It works by putting stress on muscles and bones using resistance equipment or your body weight, and they respond by growing and becoming stronger. Too much exercise over-stresses the body, but the right amount will build strength, boost energy and mood, and improve overall well-being. Lifting weights just twice a week is proven to be enough to build muscle.

No jumping required

Menopause can affect body temperature regulation. Some women notice they can't stand getting hot and sweaty or feeling uncomfortable, which can lead to avoiding exercise. The great thing about strength training is it's slow and controlled, and there's no jumping about. You take your time, tune into your body, and focus on the muscles you're moving. If you are very unfit, have reduced mobility or disabilities, you will still be able to strength train because it's easy to adapt to individual capabilities.

Always consult your doctor before starting an exercise programme. I recommend you book a few sessions with a personal trainer with relevant experience to ensure you use the correct technique and select appropriate exercises for your condition and fitness level.

Strong women stay young

Strength training has been proven to slow down and even reverse age-related muscle and bone loss. It's effective for women of all ages, including post-menopausal women who aren't taking HRT. And there appears to be no age limit. In one experiment, researchers took two groups of ninety-year-old women. One group was put on a supervised strength programme, whilst the others made no change to their daily routines. The women who did regular strength training increased bone density and muscle mass, lost body fat and improved their balance and strength. Whereas the women who didn't strength train lost bone and muscle mass, in line with natural ageing expectations.[(19)]

Strength training for metabolism

We used to think hitting menopause caused metabolism to slow down, but this isn't the case. Recent research found that the metabolism is consistent throughout adulthood until it begins to slow down from around age 60. This is a natural part of the ageing process for women and men, but we can help counter this by increasing muscle mass with strength training.

Another reason we put on weight at this age is due to reducing muscle mass and decreasing activity levels. Strength training counters this by building muscle and raising the short-term energy demands of the body. Muscles influence metabolism (the total calories we need each day), so the more muscle we have, the more calories we burn.

Build a new relationship with your body

By middle age, many women have fallen out of love with their bodies. Exercise is often viewed as a necessary evil to lose weight or compensate for overeating. No wonder we don't want to exercise when it's used as a form of punishment. However, I've seen women transform their relationships with their bodies through strength training. They fall in love with the process of becoming strong and powerful. Losing weight is less of a priority as their increasing strength and fitness become a new source of happiness. With this new respect for their body, they are more accepting of how they are. The war they've raged against their body ends, and they begin to care for themselves instead.

Exercise yourself happy

One of the great things about exercise is that some benefits are immediate. Many people notice their mood is better soon after exercising, and the effects can be felt for hours. Slow, considered exercise shifts the focus onto the present moment and steers attention towards the body. This is similar to meditation; the mind quietens and gets a rare break from thinking and worrying about everything, which in turn helps you think more clearly and rationally. Exercise spikes feel-good hormones, which explains why it lifts our mood.

Low mood, increased anxiety and depression are commonly experienced by women going through menopause. The coronavirus pandemic and unprecedented lockdowns have also taken their toll on the nation's mental health. Exercise is well-known to support mental health. It's been shown to reduce stress and anxiety and improve the quality of life of people suffering from mental health problems.[20]

Boosting your energy with exercise

Exercise is a powerful energy booster. You might feel too tired to exercise, but it's normal to feel more energetic soon after exercising, which might be surprising. When you get the level of exertion right, you'll feel better, not worse, after working out. Exercise can also help people sleep better, which raises energy levels. Many clients look forward to workouts because the improvement in energy is so transformative to their everyday life.

Whether you still have periods or not, it's normal for energy levels to fluctuate from day to day. Everyone I train, including myself feels different from week to week. It's essential to listen to your body and vary the intensity of exercise in line with how you feel. Make the most of a good day by pushing a bit harder. Then, on days when you feel tired, do fewer exercises and allow yourself to rest for longer in between.

However, there is a difference between being too tired to exercise and needing an energy boost, and it's hard to know whether working out will make you feel better or worse. When I'm feeling more tired than usual, I start my workout, and if I feel better after five minutes, I carry on. Other times, if after a few minutes I still feel like I'm fighting my body, I call it a day, knowing I need rest more than exercise. I recommend you do the same.

If you're keen to start exercising but are stressed and tired all the time, start small and build up gradually. Even 15 minutes is plenty. That way, exercise will leave you feeling energised instead of exhausted.

Poor posture and aches and pains

Many aches and pains are caused by a lack of proper movement. Modern living restricts our opportunity to move fully every day, and our bodies gradually become unbalanced. Arms and shoulders weaken if you don't regularly lift things over your head. Being hunched over a laptop tightens chest muscles pulling shoulders forward and causing neck and shoulder pain. Glutes get lazy when we sit down all day and are a common cause of lower back pain.

Working on your full-body strength through exercise can address these weaknesses and improve your posture, greatly enhancing your quality of movement and therefore, your life. That said, it's important not to self-diagnose. If you are experiencing pain, always consult your GP to rule out any serious issues and get clearance to exercise and advice on the best exercises for your condition.

What about cardio

Cardiovascular exercise is often associated with burning calories, and many weight loss programmes prioritise cardio to help with weight loss. Cardiovascular activity gets its name because it strengthens the heart, lungs and breathing muscles. This improves blood flow to the vast network of veins, arteries and tiny capillaries, which delivers blood, oxygen and nutrients deep into our tissues. It leaves skin looking brighter and may even help rebuild ageing collagen.

All exercise and activity burn calories, but many people make the mistake of thinking extra exercise is all they need. We tend to overestimate how many calories we are burning and underestimate how many we are eating. Therefore, exercise on its own is rarely an effective way to lose weight and its more effective to focus on your diet. So, rather than think about exercise as a way to burn calories or correct overeating, think about it as a way to age better. Exercise is more effective at slowing down the ageing process than anything else we can do because it has so many benefits. Studies show that as activity levels increase, the risk of death decreases. Exercise is proven to reduce the incidence of many diseases, including dementia. It improves metabolism, circulation, bone density and even the signalling between the brain and muscles.

- Strengthens heart and improves the health of arteries
- Improves lung function
- Reduces blood pressure
- Helps manage weight
- Reduces the risk of coronary heart disease and stroke
- Reduces the risk of type 2 diabetes and helps control blood sugar and insulin levels

- Reduces incidence of breast cancer in women and bowel cancer
- Reduces the risk of dementia
- Improves muscle mass and bone density
- Reduces the risk of falls

Taking even small steps to increase your general activity level is beneficial and starting small makes a difference. It's more effective to begin with 10-15 minutes of activity a day and build up gradually than do too much too soon.

The most important thing is to find something you enjoy. Brisk walking, dancing, swimming, water aerobics, cycling and jogging are all effective. The NHS recommends 150 minutes a week of moderate-intensity activity, which means exercising at a level where you can still hold a conversation. This is equivalent to around 30 minutes in total a day. It doesn't have to be done in one go either, so you could break it up into shorter sessions spread throughout the day.

Keep moving

Being inactive for long periods is now considered as bad for us as smoking. Movement Snacks are a great way to counter this by finding opportunities to move regularly throughout the day and can even burn more calories than formal exercise. It's easy to do and ideal to fit into a busy day. Set a reminder on your phone and move for a few minutes every hour.

Here are some ideas to try:

- Alternate between sitting for work and using a standing desk
- Walk around while you're on the phone

- Walk across the office to chat with colleagues instead of emailing
- Park further away from the shops
- Go up and down the stairs twice every time you go up for something
- Do a few squats or press-ups against your work surface while you're waiting for the kettle to boil
- Practice standing on one leg when you brush your teeth
- Take regular walks around your house, garden or office during work
- Do a few star jumps or jog on the spot to raise your heart rate

How much exercise should you do?

It's best to do a mixture of cardiovascular exercise and strength training. To begin with, aim for 2 x 30-minute strength training sessions with a 15-minute brisk walk each day. Start with something you can fit into your week that doesn't leave you feeling too tired, and prioritise creating a consistent routine.

As you become used to that, you may want to do more. Gradually build up to three strength training sessions a week and increase your daily walk to 30 minutes. This is a realistic amount of activity for most people and is enough for you to experience the many health benefits.

It's easy to fall into the trap of thinking more is always better, but that's not the case. When you hit the right level, you'll feel motivated and energetic. By learning to listen to your body, you'll know when it needs a rest. You're doing too much if you're achy and tired all the time, get regular sprains and strains, and feel like you have to force yourself to work out.

Common questions about strength training

Will I get too muscly?

Many women worry that they will suddenly get big muscles if they start lifting weights. But you won't. There is a difference between strength training and bodybuilding. Bodybuilders work extremely hard to achieve their physiques; it takes years of demanding training routines and eating special diets.

Will strength training help me tone up?

Yes. Strength training is the best way to tone up. When we say we want to tone up, we mean we want firmer muscles and less body fat so we can see their natural shape and contours. Strength training improves the tone and shape of your muscles, but if you want to be able to see those curves emerging, you'll need to lose body fat too.

Who Is Strength Training Suitable For?

Everyone! Whatever your age or fitness level, strength training can prevent and even reverse muscle loss. It goes without saying that before you start a new exercise programme, you should speak with your GP first.

Case studies

Savita was in her early 60s and worked full-time in her own business. By evening she was fit for nothing and could barely keep her eyes open. But, after a few months of working out for just one hour a week, she noticed a huge difference. She had more stamina and better concentration at work. More importantly, she could socialise again in the evening without falling asleep at the table! She had enough energy to get more involved with her religious community during the week, which was incredibly important to her. The only major change she'd made to her lifestyle was adding a weekly strength training session, something she'd never done before. She felt so good after each session she found herself looking for other ways to be more active during the day.

Janet was in her early 40s. Lockdown intensified an already stressful job and, as for many others, meant she sat in Zoom meetings for as long as eight hours a day. With a young family, she didn't have much spare time, so she started doing 15-minute exercise sessions three times a week. Twice before work and once at the weekend. Within just a couple of weeks, she noticed how much more energy she had and the difference it made to her concentration at work. Feeling the benefits, she was motivated to eat better and made extra efforts to be active, walking her son to school and planning weekend activities. Within a month, she'd lost a couple of kilos without really trying.

Mandy was in her 50s and came for strength training once a week. She soon noticed she had more energy, was less tired in the afternoon and slept better. After a good night's sleep, it was easier to be more active during the day, doing simple things like walking more and taking the stairs. Encouraged by her increasing energy, she started using her treadmill again. She didn't go mad, just once or twice a week in the evenings, and soon after, she added a few lunges too. Six months later, she joined a leisure club and started playing table tennis. She would have been exhausted if she'd done all this from day one. Instead, she gradually increased her activities as she felt ready, and her motivation grew as she became fitter. She slowly and naturally became more active because she enjoyed how it made her feel.

Planning and tracking progress

Print out a simple chart and use it to record progress. (See overleaf.) Ticking off workouts as you do them will motivate you to keep a routine going.

You can also record how you feel after you exercise. This can be a powerful tool for building and maintaining motivation. Here's an example of what you could track:

1. How were you feeling before your exercise?
2. How did you feel immediately afterwards?
3. How was your mood afterwards?
4. How were your energy levels?
5. How well did you sleep?
6. Was there anything else that you noticed?

If you journal regularly, you'll get a better sense of how exercise is helping you. The more you link the benefits to exercise, the more enthusiastic you'll be to keep going.

Week	Activity	Monday	Tuesday	Wednesday	Thursday	Friday	Saturday	Sunday
1	Strength	20mins		20mins		20mins		
	Cardio	15 mins walk	15 mins walk	15 mins walk	15 mins walk	Rest	15 mins walk	15 mins walk
2	Strength							
	Cardio							
3	Strength							
	Cardio							
4	Strength							
	Cardio							

Beginners' strength training workouts

You'll find the beginners' strength workouts in Part Five.

Recovery

Recovery is essential if you want the best results from your new exercise regime. A good recovery strategy means taking a break from training, getting good sleep, eating properly and even treating yourself to a massage. Exercise itself doesn't strengthen muscles. Muscles only get stronger after exercising when the body rests.

When you ache, it's because you've caused micro damage to your muscles. After this is repaired, muscles become stronger than before. Try to get a good sleep after a workout because the hormones that grow and strengthen muscles are released during deep sleep. Leaving a couple of days between workouts allows recovery to take place before the cycle starts again with your next session.

Feeding your muscles

For muscles to rebuild and repair, they need the proper nutrients. Making the connection between working out and what you eat can give you a whole new perspective on your diet. What you eat directly impacts how well you recover from exercise. Growing muscles need a regular source of complete proteins and abundant vitamins and minerals. Healthy carbohydrates deliver energy to muscles to power workouts. Following the eating principles in this book will give your body the nourishment it needs.

Hydration

Exercise can increase dehydration through sweating and faster breathing, so it's important to drink during and after working out. From a recovery point of view, water helps with muscle soreness. It transports essential nutrients into the cells to help with repair and rebuilding and flushes out toxins. Experts recommend we drink around 2 litres of water daily, yet it's easy to ignore thirst or mistake it for hunger. Caffeinated drinks, alcohol and processed, salty food increase the need for hydration. Get into the habit of drinking water rather than juices and sweetened drinks, and save the calories. A reliable sign you're well-hydrated is when your urine is pale and straw-coloured. If it's darker, increase how much you are drinking.

Massage

Massage is an incredible way to relax tight muscles and de-stress the mind. I recommend all my clients have regular massages. Those that do find themselves hooked because it becomes an essential component of their well-being and plays a vital role in enhancing their movement. Many things create tight muscles, including sitting at desks for long periods and driving. Even stress creates tension in our bodies that can tighten muscles. Stretching does help, but a qualified massage therapist will find tight muscles you didn't know you had and relax them more effectively. Massage increases blood flow to the muscles and stimulates the lymphatic system to remove waste from tissues. Human touch releases hormones that soothe us, gives us a sense of well-being, and reduces anxiety. Our muscles relax as we relax, releasing the build-up of tension they've been holding.

Find someone you feel comfortable with, and don't be shy about asking to meet them before you book. Therapists are used to seeing all body shapes and sizes, so they're not interested in what you look like. All they want to do is find those tight muscles to work on and leave you feeling relaxed. Other great options exist if you don't feel ready for a full-body massage. Face massage, Indian head massage, foot massage, and reflexology will relax and de-stress you just as well. A monthly massage is a good frequency to aim for.

Sleep

It's a fact that when we're tired, we're less able to deal with stress and more likely to make poorer food choices and eat more calories than we need. We tend to only think about diet and exercise when we want to lose weight, but if you don't sleep well and can't lose weight, that may be why.

When you're regularly sleep-deprived, cortisol levels become elevated, which is known to increase abdominal fat. Poor sleep is associated with an increased risk of weight gain, heart disease and diabetes. Adults in their 40s & 50s who sleep less than 6 hours a night are known to have an increased risk of suffering from dementia.[(21)]

Women famously struggle with sleep during menopause. Night sweats are a well-known symptom, and increased anxiety makes it difficult to switch off and harder to fall asleep. Needing to wake up to use the bathroom is also common during menopause which is another disruption to contend with.

Poor sleep can be the result of habits we've created over time. Many women find they only have a couple of hours in the evening by the time they finish their chores. They feel cheated out of precious me-time if they don't have some time to themselves before bed, but this can push bedtime back too late and leave them tired the next day. Watching TV and using phones in bed can make it harder to switch off and fall asleep.

Poor sleep is usually characterised by an inability to fall asleep quickly, waking up in the middle of the night and being unable to get back to sleep. We need between 7-9 hours of sleep a night; exactly how much is personal to you. If you're getting enough sleep, you should wake up feeling refreshed and energetic all day. If it takes a while for you to get going and you feel sleepy during the day, you're not getting enough.

Common causes of poor sleep include:

- Not giving yourself time to wind down in the evening
- Unable to quieten your mind
- Eating a heavy meal too close to bedtime
- Drinking too much caffeine during the day and especially during the afternoon
- Hot flushes and night sweats (menopause symptoms)
- Drinking alcohol before bed
- Waking up to use the bathroom
- Snoring and sleep apnoea
- Shift work
- Environment, uncomfortable bed or pillow room too hot or cold, too bright, or too noisy

Getting a good sleep every night is essential for just about every area of your life, and quality matters. There are different stages, including light, deep and REM, when we dream, and we cycle through each stage several times during the night. Each is important for different things, and deep sleep is when muscles are repaired after exercise. When you get a decent sleep, life is more manageable. Sleep improves concentration and memory and boosts the immune system. It enhances mood and the ability to cope with stress. You'll be motivated to eat well, have the discipline to give treats a miss and have enough energy to work out.

Tips for establishing a good sleep routine:

- Go to bed and get up at the same time every night, even at weekends. If you go out at the weekend, stick as close to your weekday routine as possible.
- Allow time to wind down in the evening. Put away your laptop and phone and avoid emails, addictive games, or anything that might trigger anxiety or a stress response. This includes the news or dramatic and violent TV programmes.
- Avoid working or watching TV in bed. Your bedroom should just be for sleeping or sex, which can help you relax.
- If you use a device for reading or watching TV, change the screen to a night-time setting or use blue-light-blocking glasses.
- Avoid alcohol in the evening. Whilst an alcoholic drink may help you relax and drop off to sleep, it worsens sleep quality.
- Avoid caffeine or stop drinking it in the early afternoon. Drinking coffee throughout the day can leave enough caffeine in your system to affect sleep.
- Have a relaxing bath or shower. This can help some people but may raise your body temperature if you struggle with hot flashes. If you enjoy a bath or shower before bed, don't have it too hot and give yourself plenty of time to cool down after.
- Leave 2 or 3 hours between eating and going to bed. Eating heavy, rich meals close to bedtime can interfere with sleep. On the other

hand, some people wake up hungry because blood sugar crashes. Eating a balanced evening meal with plenty of protein may help you avoid waking up hungry. Some people find a few extra carbs in the evening helps them sleep. Experiment to find the meals that best suit you.

- Being more active during the day can improve sleep. As you gradually increase exercise and activity levels, you may notice you sleep better.

Your sleeping environment

Turn your bedroom into a sleep sanctuary. Make the bed and keep the room tidy so you relax as soon as you go in.

- Use black-out blinds, heavy curtains or an eye mask to make the room as dark as possible.
- Get the temperature right. Turn radiators off or down, and leave windows open if necessary. It's better for the air to feel cool and your bed to feel cosy.
- Use an appropriate duvet tog for the season and bedding which keeps you cool and comfortable. Linen and cotton sheets are better for temperature regulation than synthetic fabrics. Duvets, pillows and mattresses made from natural fillings help with temperature regulation or look for products designed to increase airflow to keep you more relaxed at night. If you're thinking about buying a memory foam bed, do your research and check reviews. Some types retain heat and can make you overheat, waking you up at night.
- Similarly, light cotton fabrics are best if you wear clothes in bed. If you get cold feet, then bed socks will do the trick.

- Use a daylight alarm clock in a dark room. These alarms use light that gradually gets brighter to mimic dawn. They help you wake up more naturally and reduce the stress of waking up abruptly with a conventional alarm.
- Whilst phones at bedtime are mostly banned, an exception can be made for meditation apps and apps that play white noise. These can help some people fall asleep, especially if you struggle to quieten your mind.
- Try earplugs if you are disturbed by noises from your family or neighbours.

Lesser-known sleep aids

Get exposure to red light in the morning

It's not just bedtime routines that help us sleep. Getting outside early in the morning when the sun has just risen exposes us to red light. This helps reset your circadian rhythm and sends a message to your biological clock to make you feel sleepy in the evening. A short walk outside or a cup of tea in the garden within 30-60 minutes of getting up does the trick.

Try a grounding sheet

Have you ever noticed how wonderful you feel after walking barefoot on grass or sand or swimming in the sea? Until the last 150 years, humans were in constant contact with the Earth before synthetic shoes and living indoors removed that connection.

Human bodies are like electrical appliances. Electrical signals are continuously sent between our brains and bodies to allow us to navigate our environment and stay alive. Normal metabolic processes create an imbalance of positive charges, which build up, causing inflammation and damage to cells. Connecting to the Earth neutralises this charge and brings you back into balance.

Because it's not practical to stand barefoot on grass all day, grounding devices allow you to connect to the Earth from inside your home. Earthing sheets are placed on your bed and can be transformative for sleep. They connect you to the Earth via the earthing pin in UK plug sockets - they don't connect to the live pins, so you won't be electrocuted! I've had one for around a year and immediately noticed how much deeper my sleep was.

While still relatively niche, several small studies demonstrate many benefits of this simple practice. Improved sleep is one of them, as is better circulation, which can also improve the appearance of the skin, reduced inflammation, and lower anxiety levels. Grounding sheets are the perfect hack because you don't have to do anything; just lie down and close your eyes. If you are interested in learning more about this fascinating subject, check out the websites below. Both sites sell affordable grounding sheets and have plenty of scientific information on how they work. You'll also find plenty of customer reviews from enthusiastic fans, which make fascinating reading.

https://www.groundology.co.uk/
https://rowlandearthing.co.uk/

NB: I have no connection or affiliation to either of these companies.

Snoring & sleep apnoea

If you think you are spending long enough in bed but still wake up tired, you could be snoring or suffer from a serious condition called sleep apnoea. With the latter, sufferers stop breathing for short periods before momentarily waking up to take a breath. They may also make gasping, snorting and choking noises when they sleep. Sufferers don't recall these episodes, but their partners may. Snoring, although less serious, can still disturb your sleep. Being overweight, breathing through your mouth and being menopausal all increase your chance of being affected by these conditions.

Sleep apnoea puts you at greater risk of high blood pressure, stroke, difficulty concentrating at work and even having a serious accident caused by tiredness. If you suspect you may have this, speak to your GP, who will refer you to a sleep clinic for tests.

An excellent resource for snorers and sufferers of sleep apnoea is The Breathing Cure by Patrick McKeown. It explains the importance of nose breathing for good sleep and provides simple exercises to restore correct breathing during sleep so you're more alert and rested when you wake up. One of the recommendations is to tape your mouth closed while you sleep. This is less dramatic than it sounds. A postage stamp-sized piece of surgical tape is pressed lightly onto the centre of your lips to keep them together. Since reading his book a few months ago, I've adopted this practice. Admittedly I felt a bit daft at first, and I still wait until the lights are out before I put the tape on. But it's made such a significant difference I can put up with looking eccentric. I noticeably sleep deeper and more soundly and don't need to get up for the toilet as often.

When the tape is on correctly, you will still be able to talk and breathe out of the sides of your mouth. Don't use the tape if you have been drinking or are feeling unwell. If you are interested in learning more about this, visit www.oxygenadvantage.com.

Getting medical support

However, a good night's sleep continues to elude some people, whatever they try. If you are still struggling, then make an appointment with your doctor. In some circumstances, medication can be helpful, and your doctor will discuss what's available. Likewise, HRT helps many women improve their sleep. At the very least, discuss your options and make an informed choice about what route you want to take. Remember, getting good sleep each night should be one of your biggest health priorities.

Stress

Stress can significantly impact weight due to its effect on hormones and eating habits. Yet when I advise women to reduce their stress, I'm often met with resistance which is not surprising. Dealing with stress is yet another chore they don't have time for. For many, the wake-up call only comes after experiencing burnout or experiencing some life-changing event. We face up to the fact we can't cope anymore, and more significantly, we don't want to.

I didn't realise how close to burnout I was until I was fired from my job a few hours after asking my boss for support while I came to terms with my dad's terminal cancer diagnosis. Stress had been building for years, and my ability to cope had evaporated. In hindsight, I was perimenopausal, although I didn't realise it at the time. I was too busy blaming myself for being such a failure. Luckily, losing my job was the catalyst that allowed me to recover and establish a new lifestyle where I could learn to live without being controlled by relentless stress.

Balancing stress is an effective way to counter chronic stress. Our bodies are designed to switch between fight and flight mode and rest and recovery mode. You can't eliminate everything that causes stress, but you can balance it by adding more relaxation to your life. Doing things that relax you puts your body into rest and recovery mode. The more time you spend in this state, the more balanced you will be.

Reading, listening to music, watching comedy, enjoying a hobby, taking a bath, having a massage, performing gentle exercise and meditating are all stress-balancing activities. The good thing about taking this approach is that you make positive changes without needing to tackle the things that are causing you stress. To begin with, carve out a small amount of time for yourself. Even just an hour away from your responsibilities can be incredibly restorative. By experiencing the beneficial effect on your mood and energy levels, you'll be encouraged to look for other small ways to find time for yourself.

Reducing stress

There are other ways to reduce stress that take a more direct approach.

We often keep things to ourselves when we're struggling. This secrecy is something we choose, yet being open can lighten the load. One of my clients was finding her job increasingly draining. She was overwhelmed by the workload and imagined she was the only one of her colleagues who couldn't manage. Comparing herself unfavourably to the others made her feel inferior and she thought she was losing her edge. Eventually, she plucked up the courage to tell the team how she felt. To her surprise, everyone felt the same and even thanked her for bringing it up. Although it would take some time to reduce the volume of work, a colossal weight was instantly lifted from her shoulders.

Over the years, we collect responsibilities and create obligations for ourselves, becoming busier and busier. We keep going out of guilt or because we worry what others will think if we say no. The trouble is when we do more than our fair share, we become resentful. It plays on our minds as we go over our plight repeatedly. As we wind ourselves up, these imaginary conversations elevate our stress hormones.

When we ask for help, we usually get it. Friends, family and even colleagues don't want us to suffer. Unless we tell them, they won't figure it out for themselves. They're too busy dealing with their own stuff and will assume you're managing just fine.

Keeping myself busy was something I did because I thought slowing down was a sign I was getting older. I liked feeling needed and constantly looked for ways to show my family I loved them by doing things for them, which sometimes included being a busybody and getting on their nerves. It's interesting how seemingly harmless intentions can be the source of so much self-imposed pressure.

If you feel resentful about certain responsibilities, consider how you might address them. Can you just say no, delegate or do them less frequently? What's the worst thing that can happen? Sometimes, playing out a more realistic scenario of how others will respond can be helpful and give you the courage to make changes.

Learning to set boundaries and say no is incredibly liberating and powerful. Letting go of things that drain your energy frees you to discover new activities that give you joy and revitalise you. It puts you back in control of your life instead of being at the mercy of others' beck and call.

Family arguments, toxic relationships and even violent TV programmes can leave us agitated. Notice the situations that affect you and consider how you can either avoid them or handle them differently.

Having an overactive brain is incredibly common amongst women. You don't need me to tell you how draining overthinking is. But you might be surprised to know brains need an enormous amount of energy to function, as much as 20% of total daily calorie requirements.

Too much thinking isn't good for us, and scientists have established that much of our thinking is useless. Reliving an argument, playing imaginary conversations on a loop, and creating worst-case scenarios that we know will never happen. Sound familiar? Thoughts like these waste not only valuable brain power but also trigger physiological changes in our bodies. The brain can't differentiate between real and imagined threats. So, when you're catastrophising about some disaster that probably won't happen, your brain and body behave as if you are facing a genuine life and death situation.

Learning to reduce useless and destructive thoughts frees up the brain, and meditation and breathwork are effective techniques to quieten incessant overthinking. When you calm your brain, you conserve valuable mental energy and gain control over your thoughts. Instead of feeling overwhelmed and exhausted all the time, you improve your capacity to make conscious decisions when you need them. This will significantly impact your ability to stick with a healthier lifestyle long-term.

Breathwork

Breathwork is a simple practice that will quickly quieten your mind whenever you notice overthinking. It can take as little as a few minutes to calm you down. It works by shifting your attention to your breathing and activating the parts of the nervous system which put you into rest and recovery mode. Breathwork or mindful breathing is discrete, so you can do it anywhere without anyone noticing.

The way we breathe changes automatically when we experience stress. We take rapid, shallow breaths into the upper chest. It's easy to get into the habit of breathing like this throughout the day, keeping the body in fight or flight mode and elevating fat-accumulating stress hormones.

Changing how we breathe brings us back into a calm, restful state. Closing the mouth and breathing through the nose, using the diaphragm at the top of the stomach cavity to draw in the breath activates the rest and recovery mode. The more you breathe like this throughout the day, the calmer you'll feel. Try this exercise to get started.

Close your mouth and place one hand on your belly and the other on your chest. Imagine your belly button is being pulled out on a cord. As your stomach pushes out, breathe in through the nose and feel your stomach distend while your chest stays still. To exhale, pull your belly button towards your spine. Feel your stomach muscles pull in to squeeze the air back out. Repeat this a few times paying attention to your diaphragm (the muscle under your ribs). Now, allow yourself to settle into a natural breathing rhythm. Feel the air come in as the belly gently swells outwards, then let go and feel the belly relax as the air is released. Don't take deep breaths; instead, breathe lightly and gently. You can do this whenever you remember to, and before long, it will become automatic.

Anytime you feel panicked, anxious or overwhelmed, you can use this technique. After a few minutes, you'll feel calmer and better able to make conscious decisions to regain control in stressful situations.

To watch a guided video for this breathing technique, visit
www.gabrielleohare.com/book-resources

Breathwork meditation

As well as using breathwork to manage stressful situations, you can also establish a meditation practice. Regular meditation brings many emotional and physical benefits. It improves stress management, reduces negative emotions, and can increase patience and tolerance.

Ten to fifteen minutes a day is enough, to begin with. Aim to do it at the same time each day to help establish a regular routine. It's a common misconception to think you need to stop thinking to meditate. Meditation is simply about observing your thinking and noticing when your mind wanders. Instead of letting your mind get lost in a trail of thoughts, you gently bring it back to focus on the breath. To begin with, you'll be distracted by thoughts very quickly, but with regular practice, you learn to settle your thinking for longer.

Sit or lie in a comfortable position and ensure you're warm enough. Close your eyes and place one hand on your belly and the other on your chest. Take a few slow, steady breaths in and out through the nose, noticing the belly rise and fall while the chest stays still. Your mouth and jaw should feel relaxed, with your tongue lightly held against the roof of your mouth. As you breathe in, observe how your belly expands and your waist gently pushes out. Notice the cool air on the nostrils and warmer air on the back of the throat. Follow the breath as it's drawn into the stomach and as you exhale, trace it back out, noticing the light feeling of the air on your top lip as you exhale. As thoughts come up, gently take your focus back to the breath. Allow yourself to settle into a relaxed and natural breathing pattern, in and out through the nose, noticing your thoughts as they come up and letting them go again. Continue for a few minutes.

Now move your attention to your body. Slowly scan yourself from the crown of your head to your toes. Scan your forehead and scalp, around your eyes, jaw and neck. Work all the way down your body, ending at your feet. As you notice any tension, allow it to release as you breathe. Feeling fully relaxed, now return your focus to your breathing.

When you're ready to stop, wiggle your toes and fingers. Open your eyes and take your time to get up and come round.

(If you use a timer on your phone, choose a calm ring tone at a low volume so you finish the meditation gently.)

Spend some time immediately afterwards to set intentions for your day or journal while your mind is clear.

If you already have a favourite meditation practice, then continue with it. There are plenty of free and low cost meditation apps and videos online.

Managing cravings

Stress and overwhelm affect our decision-making capacity. Making a simple decision about what to have for dinner after a hectic day can easily defeat us when our brain is exhausted. Stress can trigger powerful cravings and leave us reaching for snacks to distract us from feeling uncomfortable.

Breathwork is helpful in these situations. It calms the mind so you can make conscious decisions about what to eat in line with your goals. It creates space between the urge to eat to help you identify a trigger or decide on an alternative way to deal with your emotions.

Next time you are overwhelmed by cravings or finding it hard to decide what to eat, try this exercise.

First, step away from the kitchen or the food so you are not distracted by it. Take your attention to your breath. Close your mouth and breathe in and out through your nose. If you like, you can close your eyes. Place your hand just underneath the ribs and feel the rise and fall of the diaphragm. Breathe lightly, and gently slow your breathing rate. Turn your attention away from eating and just focus on breathing and quietening your mind. As you become calmer, allow yourself to take control of the situation. Remind yourself of how you want to eat and why it matters.

If you want to eat a healthy meal, ask yourself what the best food option would be right now. If you want to resist a craving, ask yourself what you truly need right now. When you have your answers, bring yourself back into the moment, and give yourself what you need.

• PART FOUR •

CREATING CONSISTENCY

Where the Magic Happens

Consistency is where the magic happens, but it's also the most challenging part. The odd early night is great, but get a good sleep every night, and you'll feel like a new person. Swinging between healthy meals and hedonistic weekends is a guaranteed frustration trap. But commit to eating well most of the time, and you'll be relaxed about occasional indulgences, and they won't derail you.

Someone who lost over five stone once told me she never doubted she'd lose weight because inside, she was a slim person. She had put on weight during a difficult period but never lost her identity as a slim, healthy woman – even at a time when she wasn't.

We all create identities for ourselves. You weren't born a career woman or a stay-at-home mum. These were identities we chose for ourselves because it was something we wanted. It's the same with your health. If you describe yourself as a fat, lazy person who can't stop eating, your behaviour will follow. And believe me, I've often heard women describe themselves in such unkind terms. In these situations, we say we *should* be exercising or *should* be eating better, but… there's always a but. However, if you get into the habit of describing yourself as *being* something, it can increase your chance of success. For example, using phrases like, *I'm an active person*, or *I'm someone who cares about my health.* Start creating a new identity that aligns with your goals and the new behaviours you are cultivating.

As you adopt your new, healthy persona, don't hide it away. Be proud of who you are and what you stand for. Let people see you care about what you put into your body and enjoy being active. This will help you stay in control of the things you value instead of allowing your choices to be influenced by others.

We expect to learn from our mistakes in so many areas of our lives. I almost lost £50,000 for a company I worked for many years ago. When I realised what had happened, I painstakingly retraced every step until I figured out what I'd done and never made the same mistake again. Equally, when diets fail, there's always a reason, and we can retrace our steps to uncover why we found something so hard.

Our relationships with food are complicated. Many desires to eat are automatic and unconscious. Situations trigger cravings we can't resist, and we blame ourselves for being weak instead of asking what went wrong. This isn't a short-term fix, so get out of the mindset that a diet is a temporary way of eating. You're creating new, life-long habits so expect some trial and error.

Every time we start something new, we go all in, full of enthusiasm. Inevitably a time will come when, after a few consistent weeks, you hit a wall. When this happens next, which it will, resist telling yourself you've failed again. Most people catastrophise when they lose their perfect streak, but perfection is a myth and not something you should aim for. Like everyone, I have weeks when I'm in a good routine, followed by weeks when I struggle. The difference is being able to course correct without drama. When you're struck by cravings, it's an opportunity to learn something about your relationship with food, and this is a skill we can all develop.

I want to show you how powerful self-reflection is and how it can get you back on track. This is a true example of my own. For me, a good routine is eating homemade meals I enjoy, being able to last between meals without snacking, and enjoying an occasional treat. But recently, I had one of those weeks when my hunger and cravings went off the scale. Whatever I ate wasn't enough, and the cravings were so distracting I found it hard to settle and concentrate on my work. Each night I was angry with myself and vowed to get back to normal the next day, only to repeat the same pattern. After a few days of struggling, I decided enough was enough. I had to take proper control of the situation to break the cycle, and this is how I did it.

Take a step back from your emotions

When you find yourself in this position, take a step back from your emotions and look at the situation objectively. If possible, take yourself somewhere quiet and away from distractions, where you can spend some uninterrupted time reflecting.

Look beyond the food to see what's going on

When we're stuck in a food funk at the mercy of cravings, we obsess about what we've eaten and feel guilty and angry. Forget what you've eaten and change the tactic. Cravings are simply a reaction to something else.

Comparing a good week with a bad week will uncover what triggered the behaviour change.

What does a good week look like for you?

When things are going well with your eating, what does that look like for you? What are you eating? How does it make you feel, and how do you make it happen? List as many things as you can think of.

These were my answers:

- *On a good week, evening meals are planned out in advance, I know what we're having, and I stick with it during the week. On Fridays and Saturdays, I'm OK to relax a bit, and then we go back to normal on Sundays.*
- *I stick to the breakfasts that I know work well for me to keep me full*
- *I don't need to snack between meals, and I know it's because I've eaten enough for my meals*
- *I've planned lunch ahead and have time to make something proper and substantial*
- *I've got good self-control when I'm preparing food. Specifically, I'm not eating the ingredients as I'm preparing meals, e.g. munching on nuts, hacking off lumps of cheese*
- *I can surf cravings when they come up and quickly find something to distract myself and stay out of the kitchen*
- *I enjoy the food I eat and feel satisfied after it, and I don't feel the need to keep going back for more*
- *I have what I want if I go out for a meal or fancy a treat. I don't let others influence me, and I don't feel any guilt for what I choose. Consequently, I find it easy to return to my usual eating habits.*

What are the benefits of having a good week?

Next, go deeper than how you eat. How does what you eat affect your mood, energy levels and emotions?

This is what I wrote:

When I'm on top of my food, I'm mentally in a better place – simply because thinking about food takes up less space in my brain, which is incredibly freeing. I can concentrate better on my work. This makes me more productive, and because I'm getting more done, I find it easier to fit in activities that aren't work-related. I do some exercise, relax without feeling guilty and get outside for some fresh air. I'm less stressed about work, so I notice and enjoy many other things about my day, which improves my mood. My digestion is better, and I'm less bloated. My body has more time to digest food properly, so I feel lighter, balanced, and comfortable in my clothes. Wow! Even just writing this down again is a powerful reminder of the knock-on effect of good eating habits on how I feel. If this is what eating well does, why on earth can't I do this every day?

What creates a bad week?

Next, work out what the triggers might have been for your bad week. Don't write a list of what you've eaten because that's not important here. Instead, consider the events and circumstances that might have affected your routine.

This was what I noticed about my bad week:

- *I'd not slept as well as usual for two consecutive nights.*
- *The weather changed from a few weeks of mild, sunny weather to cold and rainy.*

- *Because of the weather, I'd not gone out for my usual daily walk.*
- *My HRT was mixed up after changing my prescription, and my hormones felt out of whack.*
- *I struggled with my workload and was more stressed by work, so I didn't do any exercise.*
- *My work schedule was disrupted by an unexpected situation at home which frustrated me because it meant I didn't get everything done.*
- *I felt more stressed and less relaxed overall compared to the previous weeks.*
- *My mood was lower.*

Finally, write down how this affected your eating habits

This was what I noticed:

- *Being more tired than usual, I was flagging by mid-morning and was looking for food to pick me up.*
- *By lunchtime, I felt stressed and agitated and didn't know what I wanted to eat and couldn't decide what to have. I couldn't think clearly or settle on a decision, so I just snacked on random things that I could grab quickly.*
- *I kept snacking most of the afternoon because I didn't feel like I'd had a proper lunch. (I realised I was eating less protein than usual, and I know that makes me feel hungrier)*
- *As my mood got worse, I started craving sugar and sweet things*
- *By the end of the day, I was deciding that I'd had such a bad day, I might as well make the most of it and have a treat after my dinner – and I did, but I was telling myself that it was conditional on having a good day the next day – putting pressure on the following day before it even started*

- *I felt more bloated than usual, which affected my sleep. My digestion was more sluggish, and the bloating made my mood worse and gave me more cravings.*

Interesting, isn't it? By doing exercises like these and reflecting on your eating habits, you begin to understand how circumstances affect your eating habits.

You can see from my experience how poor sleep, high workloads, low mood, and unexpected family demands easily interrupt our routines. We can't make decisions and use food as an energy and mood boost.

Course correct

The real value of this exercise is that it tells you exactly how to get back on track. As soon as I took that first step back to evaluate what was happening, the cravings and frantic eating immediately stopped. I was off the emotional rollercoaster and back in control. Then, all I needed to do was recreate a successful week. For me, this meant:

1. Going to bed earlier
2. Taking a walk before work
3. Planning substantial meals in advance for the next day

Mood and energy levels significantly impact appetite and motivation, so my first priorities were to address these. Making meal decisions the day before meant I didn't need to make decisions whilst I was hungry and stressed. I know I have fewer cravings when I eat a proper lunch, which breaks the cycle of constant snacking. Taking control and getting my day off to a positive start made me feel better, and my motivation returned.

Once you recognise a pattern, you'll likely spot it again and again. Since I first did that exercise, I've noticed the same thing happening several times. Now I better understand my weaknesses and, most importantly, know how to set myself up for a positive day.

We all go through emotional ups and downs, so it's logical to devise strategies that acknowledge them. As you become more familiar with your patterns, you'll know what you need to feel better.

Emotion	**Response**
Tiredness or low energy	Go to bed earlier Improve your wind-down routine in the evening to fall asleep faster Improve your sleeping environment Get some exercise or fresh air
Overwhelm	Plan meals in advance when you can think straight to limit decision-making when you're overwhelmed Practice meditation or breathwork to help you quieten your brain.
Low mood	Get some fresh air or exercise, or do something sociable Talk through how you feel with a partner or friend

Lack of time	Plan meals in advance Commit to exercise sessions with a friend you don't want to let down or pay for classes in advance, so you have to do it Ask for help with your workload
Stress	Practice meditation or breathwork to help you think clearly and cope better with the day's demands. Go to bed early Plan recovery and relaxation at weekends Journal or talk through how you feel with a partner or friend
Frustration	Tick off daily progress and achievements to remind yourself that you are making progress Use Journaling for self-reflection and insights into your triggers

Journaling is another effective way to cultivate self-awareness around your relationship with food. You don't need to follow a rigid structure like the one above, just find somewhere quiet and write whatever comes into your head.

Discover what works for you

While I've given you broad recommendations about how and what to eat, it's important to remember we're all individuals. The golden rule is to enjoy your food and find meals that leave you satisfied and full. When I eat something I don't enjoy, I feel cheated and crave something else to give me that pleasure hit.

I'm open to trying new ideas, but not to the extent that I'll eat things I don't enjoy just because someone else swears by them. A PT once tried to encourage me to eat smoothies for breakfast, but they didn't give me the sense I was eating something. Now and again, I'll fancy one, but I'm quickly reminded that I like chewing more than slurping.

I also know that overeating certain foods make me feel very sick. If I eat a rich dessert after a heavy meal, I often wake up in the night feeling very nauseous. I still have desserts, of course, but knowing the effect it has on me, means I make a conscious choice when I indulge and when I don't.

As you try new meals, pay attention to how they make you feel. Your goal is to discover how different foods affect you and your body. In the beginning, it can be helpful to keep a diary or journal to record how you feel after eating. Over the years, I've learned what works for me, and you'll soon do the same. Eventually, choosing to eat foods that work well for you will become second nature.

This is what I have noticed about my meals

Foods that leave me feeling full and satisfied for a long time	Foods that trigger cravings or are hard to eat in moderation	Foods that don't keep me full for very long	Foods that don't make me feel good
Full fat, high protein Greek yoghurt with berries, nuts and dark chocolate	Snacking in general, for example, when I don't make time to eat a proper lunch	Breakfast cereals	Pulses and beans can bloat me if I eat them too often
Scrambled eggs made with butter, avocado and tomato	Carb-heavy meals, e.g. pizza	Low fat, low protein natural yoghurt for breakfast	Sliced white bread & bagels give me an uncomfortable stomach ache soon after eating
Steak and salad with olive oil and balsamic dressing, and parmesan shavings	Any chocolate, sweets	Vegetarian meals (especially low-protein). Worse at lunchtime than in the evening	Very sweet, fatty foods eaten late at night (like a restaurant dessert) can make me wake up in the middle of the night feeling nauseous
Prawn or meat curry, or lentil and chickpea curry	Crisps	Light salads with fat-free dressing	Too much fruit bloats me
Vegetable soups with a side of cheese and something crunchy like oat cakes or poppadoms	Peanut butter, nut butter, nuts	High sugar fruits; bananas, apples, grapes etc.	Chinese and Indian takeaways make my face puff up

Foods that leave me feeling full and satisfied for a long time	Foods that trigger cravings or are hard to eat in moderation	Foods that don't keep me full for very long	Foods that don't make me feel good
Cheese platter with crudites and nuts (as long as it's a decent portion and not too low calorie)	Breakfast cereals	Shop-bought sandwiches and wraps	Greasy, fried foods, like bread-fried chicken or restaurant veggie burgers seem to sit in my stomach for ages and make me feel sick
Vegan chilli made filing with lentils and veg	Small meals trigger cravings soon after, whether I'm hungry or not – the little voice in my head keeps telling me I've not had enough to eat!	Smoothies as a meal. Drinking meals instead of eating them make me feel like I'm missing something	
Salads and meals with cheese added, e.g. feta in salad	Grapes	Small portions	
Scrambled eggs in butter as a snack when I've got bad cravings			
Big portions so I feel full			

Create new habits

If I had to pick the one thing that helps me eat well consistently, it would be habits. I plan meals, prepare food in advance when I know I'll be short on time later, and have the right food in the cupboards. These little routines save me many times more calories than I ever burn by exercising.

Habits, by definition, are automatic behaviours which make life easier because they reduce the number of conscious decisions we have to make. Imagine coming home from work after a stressful day to a prepared dinner. There would be no hangry arguments with yourself, or your family, about what to eat. All because you made the decision before you were tired and under pressure.

Every Saturday, I plan out the week's meals in advance and write a shopping list at the same time. I don't buy anything I don't need, just what's on my list. My teenager often complains that there's nothing nice in the house. I don't want to encourage her to snack on rubbish all the time either, but she buys her own snacks with her pocket money, so she's coping OK! The meal plan gets pinned up in the kitchen, so we all know what we're having. Depending on who finishes work first, my partner or I will make dinner. There are many times when I've been so close to ordering a takeaway after a long day. But then I realise it takes me the same time to rustle up a quick dinner, and I'll feel better the next day because of it.

Of course, we eat takeaways now and again, maybe once or twice a month, and I tend to stick to Turkish and have grilled meat and salad. My daughter has them more often, usually with her friends. If I'm honest, I'd rather she didn't, but I've found some teenager vs mum battles hard to win, and that's one of them. My tactic is to lead by example and hope that one day she can see past the allure of delivery apps and understand the importance of nutrition. I make certain that her preferences don't influence mine.

Snacking is often just another habit, and it can be helpful to think of it that way. Maybe you aren't a sugar addict after all; you just got into eating sweet things. To break a bad habit, you need to disrupt the routine. Look for the action that triggers the craving and change it. If having a cup of tea makes you want a couple of biscuits, or you can't walk past your favourite coffee shop without ordering a latte, switch to coffee, or take a different route.

Track your progress

Another worthwhile habit is tracking your progress. Make it more than a weekly weigh-in and use it to learn about your habits, triggers, and preferences. This will help you build a stronger connection between what you eat and how you feel. As you make changes, pay attention to energy levels, sleep, mood, digestion, cravings and hunger. Notice which meals work best for you and your family, and ditch the ones that don't hit the spot. The more positive changes you notice, the more motivated you'll feel.

When things don't go to plan, get curious instead of discouraged. And remember to practice compassion! Instead of beating yourself up when you succumb to temptation or feel overwhelmed by cravings, try uncovering what's happening. Acknowledge when obstacles crop up, observe how you react to them, and see if you can spot any patterns. The more you understand your relationship with food, the better equipped you'll be to improve it.

Here's a suggested format for tracking your progress. Aim to do it weekly to remind yourself about your primary goal and set smaller actions for that week. If weighing yourself triggers you, then don't do it. You can take measurements or just go by how clothes fit or feel. Health and well-being are more than a number on a scale, so find the things that motivate rather than discourage you.

Weekly Progress Tracking		
My overall goal is:		
This week's goal is:		
My key actions to hit this week's goal are:		
Progress Tracking	**This week (vs last week)**	**Comments/Observations**
Weight		
Measurements		
Exercise		
Energy levels		
Sleep		
Mood		
Digestion		
Stress/Anxiety		
Other		

What's worked well this week?
What's been challenging this week?
What can I improve on next week?
What is my goal for next week?
How will I feel when I hit that goal?
How will I reward myself for achieving it?

Trust the process

Changing your weight for good means improving your diet, exercising regularly, managing stress, and getting enough sleep. All parts of the process are important. If you're constantly challenging it, making excuses, and creating exceptions to the rules, you'll erode the effectiveness of the approach. Sometimes, when we're determined to lose weight, we fixate on calorie restriction and exercise. We dismiss advice on stress management, sleep, and recovery, even when weight loss stalls. Stay open to all areas of the approach and gradually make improvements in each. Often, the things we resist are the very things we need to work on.

Reward yourself

Changing your diet and building an exercise habit takes time and effort. We rarely reward ourselves for the lengths we go to and, in doing so, miss out on a vital source of motivation. Reward tactics work, which is why they are commonly used at work and with children, but I bet you rarely think about rewarding yourself.

Rewards strengthen the link between the work required to achieve a goal and the goal itself. They are used to boost motivation and drive to do the hard work. So, if you're putting yourself under pressure to work harder, make sure you get rewards too! Decide on key milestones and allocate an appropriate reward Milestones can be significant, like losing half a stone or small, such as exercising three times in one week. Simple rewards like putting a £1 coin in a jar each time you work out can be just as effective as booking yourself a massage when you lose half a stone. Make sure to plan rewards in advance and follow through when you hit your milestone. It's OK to use food as a reward now and again, but it's better to find different experiences you enjoy.

Make your environment work for you

If your cupboards are full of processed foods you can't resist, you're going to eat them. If you don't have the ingredients you need to make an enjoyable, healthy meal, you'll go back to your old staples. The food environment we live in profoundly affects how we eat. Adapting your environment sets you up for success if you are serious about your goals.

Otherwise, you'll quickly be defeated if you're continually fighting clutter and temptation.

If you're a snacker, like me, don't make it easy to grab foods without thinking. Remember my client with the jar of nuts on her counter? Now she keeps them near the back of a high cupboard. She mostly forgets about them, and if she does fancy one, she can't be bothered to get them out.

I cleared out a little cupboard for my daughter and buy her things so she can make her own meals if she doesn't fancy what I'm making. She was away with her dad when I first did it. I filled it with a few basics like pasta and pesto, baked beans, crackers, some crisps and chocolate, decaf coffee, peanut butter, cashews, tins of tuna and a few fun things. I sent her a photo of it, and she loved it – to the extent she even posted it to her friends, a seal of approval for sure! It's worked better than I expected and has encouraged her to be more independent with her cooking, which means less work for me. I can keep my cupboards full of the food I want to eat, and don't face temptation each time I open the door.

Apply a similar approach to other areas of your home. You will sleep far better in a relaxing, tidy room with comfortable bedding and black-out blinds than in a room piled high with ironing, a massive TV and flimsy curtains.

One of my clients cleared out a small corner of her lounge so she could exercise and laid out an exercise mat and a few weights. She allocated a time to work out before the family came in to watch TV in the evening, and it worked brilliantly. If you plan to walk every day, buy a waterproof coat so rainy weather can't stop you. Remove as many barriers as possible between you and your goals to make it effortless and automatic to incorporate the new behaviours you want to adopt. Tie your environment into your new identity as a health-loving person. Figure out what it will take to create your new lifestyle, then adapt your home to facilitate it.

Connection

Connection also has a significant role to play in long-term success. It takes time to make new habits automatic and overcome challenges. Because women have such a unique experience to dieting and have different motivations as we hit our forties (and beyond), I'd like to invite all readers to join my free, private Facebook group, so we can continue our journeys together and support each other along the way.

To join, visit
www.gabrielleohare.com/book-resources

Final Words

Learning to listen to your body

Our bodies are amazing. We are all born with a sense of intuition because our brains are connected to millions of tiny sensors reacting to both the external environment and our internal state, constantly working to keep us in balance. Our body can communicate with our conscious mind, to tell us what it needs. We just need to listen.

One of my clients told me that whenever things kick off at work, she has to go for a run to burn off stress. This is an effective, natural way to deal with the build-up of intense pressure. When I'm writing, and my concentration dips and my brain gets cloudy, I let my brain rest instead of trying to force it. After a break, I come back fresher, with a different perspective and start making progress again. Some days I feel unusually tired, and have no problem having an afternoon nap if I can fit one in. I'm done with trying to struggle stubbornly through the day and am learning to give my body what it needs

Listening to your body can improve your relationship with food. Mindful eating is a simple practice which helps restore our connection with food and re-educate our appetites. It's used as a natural way to control weight based on the premise that if we only eat when we are hungry and stop when we are full, we gradually return to our ideal weight.

As you become used to eating healthier meals, you may also be interested in practising mindful eating. You start by learning to experience true hunger. True hunger is characterised by a growling stomach and a distinct sensation of emptiness, which gradually intensifies until it's impossible to ignore, a sign you're ready to eat.

Mindful eating includes using all your senses as you eat and taking time to notice the aromas, the colours, and even the presentation, which adds to the anticipation. When your mouth waters, it signals the digestive process is starting. As you take your first bite, you pay attention to the taste and texture. Each mouthful is thoroughly chewed, which also improves digestion. As you continue to eat, you tune into how the taste of the food changes. With genuine hunger, the first few mouthfuls taste amazing, whatever you are eating. As you continue to eat, tastebuds become less sensitive, and you lose interest in the food. This is accompanied by a sensation of fullness, which becomes uncomfortable. These are the signals to stop eating because your energy and nutrition needs have been met.

This is how hunger hormones connect with our senses and instinct to regulate food intake, so we don't eat more than we need. Yet, many of us no longer register these sensations. We eat before we feel hungry and carry on well past the point of enjoyment, overloading our digestive systems in the process. No wonder so many of us suffer from bloating and digestive issues.

Another benefit to mindful eating is that it helps you identify which foods satisfy you the most and make you feel fuller for longer. This allows you to make smarter choices when deciding what to eat. Mindful eating principles also teach us to eat treats in moderation, which is crucial because we can't escape them. There's no reason why they can't be a regular part of your diet as long as you make conscious decisions to eat them, and don't let emotional eating and cravings take control or allow bad habits to creep back in. This may sound alarming when you've been used to avoiding certain foods for years. We imagine if we allow them back into our diets, we'll go overboard, yet that's not always the case. When foods aren't forbidden, they lose their appeal. It becomes easier to manage cravings and eat smaller amounts less regularly.

Mindful eating does take some practice to retrain yourself to eat only when hungry and stop when you are full. You will gradually achieve your natural, ideal weight once you can do this. It can be a sustainable long-term weight maintenance method because it is less restrictive than many diets and therefore easier to live with.

Practice self-acceptance and body positivity

Dieting has long been associated with achieving a perfect body. Unless we are mindful of the process, it can lead to obsessing over perceived imperfections and directing a lot of self-hate towards ourselves for falling short of idealised body standards. I don't believe we should feel pressured to look a certain way, be judged or feel less-than because of our weight and body type. I certainly don't subscribe to the ideals of perfect bikini bodies.

I've written this book because stressful, modern living combined with an increasingly unhealthy food environment has disconnected us from our appetites. Over the years, this has taken its toll on our health and well-being. Many people don't understand why they become overweight and feel powerless to change it. The idea that our weight is at the mercy of external factors and is outside our control is horrifying. Worse, we tend to mistakenly blame ourselves, which creates low self-esteem and a lack of confidence.

Eating nutritious foods, moving your body and getting adequate rest are all ways to be kind to yourself. The benefits extend way beyond simply reducing a number on a scale. As you gradually improve your lifestyle, remember healthy, beautiful bodies come in all shapes and sizes. The confidence radiating from within us, our smiles, our posture, our energy and our zest for life says more about who we really are than a comparison to a photoshopped supermodel ever could.

Be compassionate to yourself at all times

We are unkinder towards ourselves than anyone else. Imagine if your friend, partner, or child spoke to you the same way you talk to yourself. You'd be distraught! We judge ourselves especially harshly when we diet. We expect to achieve impossibly high standards and are heavily critical when we fall short. We blame ourselves for being lazy and unmotivated. Yet as we've seen, we only fail because we're so busy looking after everyone else.

We need to be compassionate because change is tough, even more so when you're stressed and menopausal. Practising self-compassion is critical if you want to succeed this time because it breaks the pattern of previous dieting attempts.

At its simplest, compassion means accepting some days will feel harder than others. When you notice you're struggling, lean into it and find the cause. Use journaling and breathwork to discover your triggers and take back control. Reach out to your community to get support and encouragement to stay with it.

Another example of being unkind to yourself is falling into the trap of denying yourself anything and everything until you've reached your goal. I've heard stories of women who spend as little as possible on nice clothes because they don't want to waste their money on dressing a body they don't like. They live in the hope that one day they will be a different size, but that day never comes. Instead, they force themselves to wear clothes they don't feel good in and end up feeling even worse, often turning back to food for comfort.

Take the opposite approach and show yourself compassion by being your cheerleader. Celebrate yourself today as you are now. Don't allow yourself to only fixate on what you have or haven't eaten; instead, do as many things as possible to make yourself feel loved and appreciated. Buy something new to wear or brighten up old favourites with new accessories. Replace worn-out underwear and treat yourself to a facial or a massage. Make time to style your hair, update your make-up, and get the perfume out. Treating yourself like this is powerful. It makes you feel better because it reminds you that you are worth the effort. Constantly show yourself kindness and respect, and you'll tune into what makes you feel good and realise how little effort it takes. You'll feel happier, more relaxed, and better able to deal with life's pressures.

Small changes like this can trigger other changes. Start being kind to yourself by doing anything that makes you feel good. The boost you get will fire up your motivation enough to get you thinking about what else you can do for yourself.

Take ownership of pleasure in your life

We all need more pleasure in our lives. Without pleasure, chores become a burden, and we feel down and resentful. Women work incredibly hard, yet we are often taken for granted, and children, partners, and bosses rarely show us the appreciation we deserve.

Pleasure is an essential reward for hard work that directly affects motivation levels. Menopause further dulls the ability to experience pleasure, which is why motivation plummets around this time. Losing your get-up-and-go and your drive to get things done sucks. Finding ways to bring more pleasure into your life helps counter this, making you feel better in yourself and reigniting your spark.

For many, food has become a primary source of pleasure. With little time to ourselves and too much on our minds, we turn to food because it's convenient and takes no effort. Lose the reliance on food as a mood-booster and build a wider repertoire of things that make you feel good. Reward yourself for hard work, hitting milestones and achievements. Use small, frequent gestures to continually show your appreciation for the effort you put into each day.

Bringing pleasure back into our lives is essential, and we must take responsibility for giving pleasure to ourselves. We can't rely on others for this. Pleasure feeds motivation. If we want to be motivated to do the extra work that comes with overhauling our health, we must find a way to weave pleasure into everyday life by rediscovering the things that bring us joy.

Settle for less than perfection

We know perfection doesn't exist, yet we place enormous demands on ourselves to achieve it. One reason we fail is when our day doesn't go to plan; we eat something 'bad' or miss a workout. The loss of control and losing our streak of good days frustrates us, leading to self-sabotage and eventually abandoning our diet. Many clients return to training after a holiday, feeling sheepish about what they've eaten or apologetic because they've eaten a slice of their child's birthday cake. There is room to eat for pleasure and celebrations and to break the monotony of routines. Learning to accept this rather than feeling guilty all the time is genuinely liberating.

You've heard of the saying, where attention flows, energy goes. Put your time and effort into improving the quality of the food you eat each day rather than obsessing or feeling guilty about the occasional indulgences.

It's your time now

Our happiness and the quality of our lives aren't measured by the bathroom scales. And whilst nutrition and exercise can reduce your weight, the real power lies in their ability to do so much more. I hope this book has given you a new perspective on how to use food, exercise, sleep, and stress management as stepping-stones to whatever dreams you have for the future. This is your time.

• PART FIVE •

RESOURCES

Recipes

Making regular, home-cooked, balanced meals is less work than you think. Here are some quick and easy recipes I use at home to get you started and give you some ideas. There are far better cooks out there than me, but these have worked well for my family over the years. Having a small repertoire of meals I can cook on repeat, makes life easier and saves time and money.

When I first wrote out these recipes to give my clients, I was surprised by how low-calorie they were. It just goes to show how home-cooked meals help you stay slimmer. Don't stop with these recipes; keep experimenting until you find the ones that work for you and your family.

BREAKFASTS

Yoghurt, Berries & Nuts

Serves 1 Approx. calories 334

A quick and simple breakfast and surprisingly filling. The key is to use full-fat yoghurt. I use 10% fat Greek yoghurt, which is higher in protein than other types. Nuts boost the protein content, and the combination of protein and healthy fats keeps you full.

TIP: Use warm berries in winter for a comforting start

150g Full Fat Greek Yoghurt
80g mixed berries (I use frozen, which are great value for money)
25g mixed nuts (any type)
Mix together and serve.

Buckwheat Pancakes

Serves 1: Approx. calories 414

Buckwheat is a complete protein so great for vegetarians; it's also gluten-free. If you prefer, you can swap for the same weight of oats, self-raising flour (omit the baking powder) or gluten-free flour. You'll need a blender to achieve a smooth batter if you're using oats.

Pancake Mix

40g buckwheat flour (or alternative)
1 medium egg
Approx. 75ml milk or dairy-free alternative 1/2 tsp baking powder
Pinch salt
5g butter for frying

Topping

50g berries
30g Greek yoghurt, or dairy-free alternative
20g mixed seeds (e.g. chia, pumpkin) Sprinkling of cinnamon (optional)

Mix together to a smooth batter about the consistency of thick, double cream.

Heat the butter in a non-stick pan and pour the batter into the pan to make one big pancake or smaller ones.

Leave until bubbles appear on the top and check to see if the underside of the pancake is brown.

Flip over and cook the other side until golden.

Top with the fruit, yoghurt & seeds and serve.

Chocolate Smoothie

Serves 1: Approx. calories 309

Freeze bananas into chunks and take them out of the freezer as you need them. It makes the smoothie colder, too, which I prefer.

1/2 a medium banana
1 scoop of protein powder or 75g full-fat Greek yoghurt or vegan alternative
1/2 avocado
1 heaped tsp cocoa powder
150g milk or dairy-free milk

Blend everything together and serve immediately.

Chia & Blueberry Pot

Serves 1: Approx. calories 327

A plant-based breakfast that can be made the night before. If you make it in the morning, you will need to let it stand in the fridge for 10-20 minutes to let the chia seeds absorb the liquid.

15g Chia Seeds
80g blueberries (defrosted if using frozen)
20g mixed nuts (any type)
100 ml Almond milk (or any dairy-free milk)
50g Coconut Yoghurt (or any plain dairy-free alternative)

Mix together and serve.

Eggs & Mushrooms

Serves 1: Approx. calories 270

3 medium eggs
10g butter for frying
A handful of mushrooms and/or spinach

Fry mushrooms and spinach in half the butter until soft, remove from the pan and keep warm. Wipe the pan, then add the remaining butter. Fry or scramble the eggs, depending on what you prefer. When cooked, add the veg and serve.

Optional: Add a slice of rye bread + 125 calories, or 3 oatcakes +144 calories

Bacon & Mushrooms

Serves 1 : Approx. calories 270

3 rashers of back bacon
5g butter for frying
A handful of mushrooms and/or spinach

Place the bacon under the grill and melt the butter in a small frying pan. Fry the veg until soft, then keep warm until the bacon is cooked. Plate everything together and serve.

Optional: Add a slice of rye bread + 125 calories, or 3 oatcakes +144 calories

Berry Smoothie

Serves 1: Approx. calories 380

250ml full-fat milk or vegan alternative
80g berries of choice (frozen or fresh)
1 small banana
75g full-fat Greek yoghurt or dairy-free alternative

Optional: 1 tbs oats +56 cals

Scrambled Egg, Avocado & Tomato

Serves 1: Approx. 358 calories

3 medium eggs
1/2 medium avocado, sliced
1 medium tomato sliced
5g butter
Salt & pepper to taste
1 tsp olive oil (optional)

Beat the eggs together and season. Melt the butter in a frying pan and scramble the eggs. When cooked, serve with the avocado and tomato and season to taste.

Optional: drizzle the olive oil over the avocado

Smoked Salmon & Cream Cheese on Rye

Serves 1: Approx. calories 388

50g smoked salmon
1 piece of rye bread (you can also use a medium slice of sourdough or other GF bread. Just keep it to one slice!)
25g full-fat cream cheese (e.g. Philadelphia)
Lemon and black pepper to season

Lightly toast the rye bread on both sides. Spread with the cream cheese and lay the smoked salmon on top. Season with lemon and black pepper and serve.

LIGHT MEALS

Make lunch a proper meal to keep you full for longer and avoid afternoon energy crashes.

Mackerel & Feta Salad

Serves 1: Approx. calories 455

The ready filleted versions work well and are quick to prepare. If you don't like mackerel, swap for smoked salmon or trout.

1 prepacked mackerel fillet (approx. 80g weight) 30g feta cubed
Large serving of mixed salad; e.g. lettuce
Radish
Olives
Cucumber
Beetroot
10 ml olive oil for the salad (or tablespoon of mayo)
Vinegar or lemon to dress the salad and fish.

Arrange everything on a large plate and serve.

Greek Salad

Serves 1: Approx. calories 415

Very quick and easy to make. Not skimping on the cheese makes this very filling.

100g feta cubed
5 cherry tomatoes halved
10cm piece cucumber diced
Half a red or green pepper diced
10 black olives in brine
Mixed leaves (optional)
A pinch of dried oregano or mixed herbs to finish
10 ml olive oil, lemon juice or vinegar of your choice

Arrange everything on a large plate and serve.

Spinach & Feta Omelette

Serves 1: Approx. calories 415

You can put any mix of veg in your omelette. Mushroom, peppers, red onion, frozen peas or beans work well. The difference in calories will be minimal. I use frozen spinach, which makes it very convenient. Use about 3-4 cubes. Defrost them first and squeeze as much water out as possible.

3 eggs lightly beaten
Salt & pepper to taste
30g feta cubed
2-3 cubes of frozen spinach, defrosted and all water squeezed out
5g butter for frying
Large serving of mixed salad; e.g. Lettuce, Radish, Cucumber, tomato, pepper, spring onion
10 ml olive oil for the salad (or tablespoon of mayo)

Mix the drained spinach and feta into the beaten egg and season with salt and pepper to taste. Melt the butter in a frying pan and tip the mixture into it. Cook on a medium to low heat until the mixture is just cooked all the way through. Finish by browning the top under a grill. Serve with the dressed salad.

Bacon, Feta & Broccoli Warm Salad

Serves 1: Approx. calories 480

A handy dish for using up random leftovers in the fridge. I always have bags of frozen beans, peas, broad beans and spinach in the freezer, which are useful for adding bulk to leftovers.

2 rashers of back bacon chopped into pieces
30g feta cubed
80g broccoli
80g of frozen veg (e.g. peas, beans, broad beans)
10ml olive oil
10g walnuts chopped into large pieces
Optional: Mixed leaves to serve
Salt & pepper to taste.

Boil the broccoli until nearly tender, then add the frozen veg into the pan for the last couple of minutes. Drain any excess water and keep warm. Dry fry the bacon in a frying pan until brown. Add the chopped walnuts to the bacon and warm through for a minute or so. Tip the drained veg into the pan, add the olive oil and mix everything together. Add the feta last and mix gently. Season to taste and serve.

Haloumi & Chickpea Salad with Tzatziki

Serves 1: Approx. calories 560

A very substantial salad which will keep you full until your next meal.

100g sliced halloumi

Chickpea Salad

50g tinned chickpeas drained
2 tsp olive oil
Juice of half lemon plus a few gratings of the lemon peel
1 tbs chopped coriander
Salt & pepper to taste
Mixed salad, e.g. lettuce, tomato, radish, pepper etc.

Tzatziki

Use shop-bought, or to make your own, stir diced cucumber into 50g Greek yoghurt. Add a pinch of salt, a squeeze of lemon and a good pinch of dried mint. Stir together.

Make the chickpea salad by mixing all the ingredients together. Grill the halloumi until golden.

Serve with the chickpea salad and the mixed green salad. Add the tzatziki and serve.

Sweet Potato & Smoked Salmon Frittata

Serves 1: Approx. calories 457

3 medium eggs beaten
Salt and pepper
5g butter
1/2 small red onion
100g cooked sweet potato cut into cubes
50g smoked salmon
Large serving of mixed salad.
10ml olive oil and vinegar to dress the salad.

Fry the onion in the butter until soft, then tip into the beaten egg. Tip the sweet potato into the beaten egg, season well and mix together. Tip everything back into the pan and set over a medium heat until the egg is firming up. Lay the smoked salmon slices across the top and finish under the grill.

Spanish Salad

Serves 1: Approx. calories 386

Based on the ubiquitous side salad in Spain, with the addition of new potatoes to make it a more substantial meal.

1 medium hard-boiled egg
1 tin tuna in brine, drained
4-5 small boiled new potatoes
1 tbs tinned or frozen sweetcorn (defrosted)
5 olives, sliced
3 anchovy fillets in oil, drained (optional)
A few slices of red onion
A couple of handfuls of chopped iceberg lettuce
10ml olive oil and white wine vinegar to dress
Salt & pepper to taste

Arrange everything on a large plate and serve

Hummus & Crudites

Serves 1: Approx. 450 calories

100g shop-bought hummus
10 olives
Chopped raw veg, e.g. cucumber, radish, carrot, pepper, celery
3 oatcakes

Arrange the vegetable crudites and oatcakes on a plate and serve with the hummus.

Omelette

Serves 1: Approx. 381 calories

3 medium eggs
10g butter for frying
Approx. 100-150g mixed veg, e.g. Peppers, mushroom, onion, spinach
15g grated cheddar
Mixed salad

Melt half the butter in a non-stick frying pan and saute the veg until soft. If using spinach, add it last and drain any water that is released. Beat the eggs and season to taste. Add the cooked veg to the egg mixture and stir to mix in. Wipe the pan, melt the remaining butter, and then tip in the egg mixture. Cook until the egg is just cooked through. Add the grated cheese to the top, then place under a hot grill to melt. Serve with a mixed salad.

Tuna Mayo

Serves 1: Approx. calories 320

1 Tin tuna in brine or spring water, drained
2 tsp mayonnaise
Small handful of finely chopped crunchy veg, e.g. pepper, cucumber, radish, spring onions
5 olives, sliced
1tsp capers (optional)
Green salad

Mix everything together and serve with the green salad

Optional: Pitta bread +160 calories, 150g Baked sweet potato +130 calories, 3 oatcakes +144 calories

Tuna Niçoise Salad

Serves 1: Approx. 350 calories

120g Tinned Tuna in brine or spring water, drained
10 olives
2-3 Anchovies
1 Tsp Capers
80g steamed green beans
Mixed salad leaves

Dressing: 15ml olive oil, 1/2 tsp Dijon mustard, 10ml white wine vinegar

Optional: 100g boiled potatoes + 110 calories

Italian Tagliata

Serves 1: Approx. 357 calories

120g Sliced cooked beef or steak (trimmed of fat)
15g shaved parmesan cheese
Mixed lettuce leaves and/or rocket
80g cherry tomatoes halved
15ml olive oil
20ml Balsamic vinegar reduced by half in a small pan

Arrange lettuce, rocket and tomatoes on a plate and scatter shaved parmesan over the top. Place the sliced beef over the top of the salad. Pour the balsamic vinegar into a small pan and bring to the boil to reduce it by half; this won't take long. Add the olive oil to the reduced balsamic and mix. Pour over the beef and serve.

Optional: 100g boiled potatoes +110 calories

Cheese & Nut Platter

Serves 1: Approx. 439 calories

A simple, tasty lunch that takes no time to prepare.
60g Sliced cheese of choice
25g Mixed nuts
Veg crudites
Mixed salad

Optional: 3 oatcakes + 144 calories

Arrange the cheese on a plate and serve with the nuts, crudites and salad, and the oatcakes if using.

Mackerel Pate

Serves 1: Approx. 450 calories

120g smoked mackerel fillets (skin & bones removed)
Grated rind and juice of ½ a lemon
1tsp capers (optional)
1 tsp mayonnaise
Salt and pepper
Crudites, e.g., cucumber, celery, pepper, radish

Using a blender, process the mackerel with the rest of the ingredients and mix until smooth. Alternatively, mash together until everything is combined. Season to taste. Serve with salad & crudites

Tuna & Olive Pate

Serves 1: Approx. 288 calories

120g tin tuna in brine or spring water, drained weight
85g black olives in brine, drained
1 tsp mayo
Lemon juice to taste and to loosen pate to desired consistency
Crudites, e.g., celery, little gem lettuce leaves, radish, pepper
Mixed leaves

Add the tuna, olives and mayonnaise into a processor and process until smooth. Add lemon juice as desired to get the preferred consistency. Season to taste. Serve with salad and crudites.

Optional: 3 oatcakes +144 cals, medium pitta + 160 cals

Chicken Soup

Serves 1: Approx. calories 440

1 medium leek, sliced
1 tsp butter
200ml chicken stock
100g potato peeled and diced
50g frozen peas
120g cooked and chopped chicken breast
Salt and pepper

Soften the leek in a large pan in 1 tsp butter. Add the chicken stock and potato. Bring to the boil and simmer until the potato is cooked. Add the chicken breast and frozen peas. Bring everything back to the boil and simmer for 10 minutes until the chicken and peas are piping hot. Season with salt and pepper to taste.

For more meat-free lunch ideas, see 'Making Vegetables the Main Event'.

MAIN MEALS

Keep meals simple by basing them on protein and veg. Carbs can be added individually according to preference and appetite. Double up portions and freeze for later in the week, or eat the following day for an instant, filling lunch that will keep your energy levels consistent all afternoon.

Prawn Curry and Poppadoms

Serves 2: Approx. calories 416

Use the same recipe and swap out the prawns for any meat, a tin of chickpeas, paneer or halloumi cheese. (Calories will vary). Add rice or shop-bought naan bread if making for the rest of the family.

Curry

250g fresh or frozen prawns (defrosted according to package instructions)
1 clove chopped garlic
2 tsp coconut oil
2 tbs tomato puree
2 tsp curry powder
1 tsp cumin powder (or extra tsp of curry powder)
Chill powder to taste
Salt and pepper
1-2 tbs chopped coriander & finely sliced ginger to garnish
2 microwave poppadoms

Raita

Mix one finely chopped tomato and a 2-inch slice of cucumber diced. Mix together and add a pinch of salt, a squeeze of lemon and 1tbs chopped coriander.

Yoghurt sauce

Stir 1/2 tsp dried mint into 50g Greek yoghurt. Add a pinch of salt and a pinch of cumin, and a squeeze of lemon. Mix together and thin with a splash of milk if desired.

In a large non-stick frying pan, fry the garlic in oil until soft. Add the spices and tomato puree and fry in oil for a few minutes to get a curry paste. Gradually add water to the pan and stir until you get a sauce-like consistency; bring to the boil and simmer for 20 minutes. Watch carefully as you want the sauce quite thick. Add a lid to the pan if it splutters and keep an eye on the sauce to make sure it doesn't catch. Add the prawns, which should thin the sauce out slightly. Add a splash of water if needed. Bring back to the boil and simmer until prawns are cooked through. Add salt & pepper to taste and finish with chopped coriander. Serve with the Raita, yoghurt sauce and 2 microwave poppadoms.

Paella

You don't need to avoid carbs; just eat fewer overall. We are simply in the habit of basing all meals around carbohydrates. In this plan, we're switching that around to focus more on protein and small amounts of healthy fats. Meals with more carbs (like this one) are great to have on days when you work out or are more active than usual.

Serves 2: Approx. calories per portion 500 (without mayo)

100g chorizo, cubed (from a chorizo ring)
1 red or yellow pepper sliced
175g of frozen seafood selection (prawns, squid and mussels) or frozen prawns if you prefer, defrosted according to package instructions
100g arborio rice
200ml boiling water
1 rounded tsp smoked paprika
1/2 tsp dried oregano
Large pinch of saffron (optional)
80g frozen beans
Salt & pepper to taste
Lemon wedges to serve
Mixed salad to serve

Optional: Aioli (fresh garlic grated into mayo)

Dry fry the chorizo in a frying pan until lightly browned on a medium to low heat. As the sausage releases its oil, use a paper towel to soak up the excess. When browned on both sides, leave a small amount of oil in the pan, add the pepper, and stir fry for 5-8 minutes until softened. Add the rice and spices to the pan and stir to coat in the oil, herbs, and spices for 2-3 minutes. Add the water to the pan and stir briefly. Bring to the boil, then simmer for 20-30 minutes. Stir occasionally to check the rice isn't sticking and gradually add more water if needed allowing it to absorb. Repeat until the rice is soft, and the liquid is absorbed. Add the seafood, green beans and saffron, and turn up the heat to bring back to the boil to heat everything through until it is piping hot. Add a splash of water if the mixture starts to catch. Season to taste and serve with lemon and a mixed salad.

Cod & Parma Ham

Serves 1. Approx. calories 490

150g cod fillet
2 slices of Parma ham
80g of mixed frozen veg (beans, peas, broad beans)
One medium-large tomato chopped
1 tablespoon of canned green lentils, drained.
10ml olive oil
Vinegar of your choice to taste
Chopped tarragon (optional)
Salt & pepper to taste
80g new potatoes
1-2 tsp pesto (optional)

Wrap the cod in the Parma ham and cook in the oven at 180 until cooked through. Defrost the frozen veg in boiling water for a few minutes. Drain well, then mix in the lentils, tomatoes and tarragon if using. Add the oil, vinegar, salt, and pepper to taste and keep warm until everything is ready. Boil the potatoes until tender, add the pesto if using and mix well. Plate the fish, vegetables and potatoes and enjoy.

Salmon & Pesto Potatoes

Serves 1: Approx. calories 384

Frozen wild salmon filets are available at most supermarkets and are convenient and economical. Use fresh salmon if you prefer.

150g salmon
20g sliced onion marinated in salt and lemon for 10 minutes
100g frozen vegetable (e.g. beans, peas, broad beans)
4 radishes sliced
100g new potatoes
1-2 tsp pesto
10ml olive oil
Vinegar to taste
Salt & pepper to taste

Roast salmon in the oven until cooked, according to instructions on the packaging. Finely slice the onions and place them in a medium-sized bowl that will fit all of the veg in. Marinade the onions in a large pinch of salt and squeeze of lemon juice for 10-15 minutes or while you cook the salmon and the potatoes. This will soften the texture and the flavour. Slice the radish and tip on top of the onions. Don't mix in. Defrost the veg in boiling water and heat through until just cooked and tender. Drain well and add to the bowl with the onions and radish. Add oil, vinegar, salt and pepper to taste and mix everything together. Boil the potatoes until cooked, then mix with the pesto. When the salmon is cooked, serve with potatoes and vegetables.

Steak & Black Bean Salad

Serves 1: Approx. calories 440

1 x medium steak approx. 150g (whichever type you prefer, excess fat removed)
1/2 tin black beans
1/4 finely chopped onion
1tbs chopped coriander
Approx. 5cm finely chopped cucumber
2 medium tomatoes, seeds removed and chopped finely
Juice of 1/2 lime
½ tbs olive oil
Chopped chilli or chilli flakes to taste
Salt & pepper to taste

Cook steaks to your preference and slice them into strips. Mix the black bean salad ingredients together and adjust the seasoning to taste

Optional Extras:

Adding grated cheese and shop-bought tomato salsa also works well and doesn't add many calories to the meal.

1 Tbs Grated cheese + 62 cals Tbs Salsa + 20 cals

If you are cooking this for others in your family, serve with tortillas or pitta (check packaging for calories)

Bolognese

Serves 4: Approx. calories per portion 400

Bolognese sauce is a staple in my household. It's a classic example of a meal that is traditionally served with a big portion of carbs, yet it works brilliantly without. If making for the rest of the family, give them the option of having pasta. If you want pasta with yours, that's fine, just have more sauce and less pasta to keep the calories/carbs down and make it more filling.

500g beef mince (calories based on 15% fat, use lower fat if available)
1 onion chopped
1 clove chopped garlic
1 carrot chopped
1 tbs olive oil
2 tins chopped tomatoes
2 tbs tomato puree
100g mushrooms sliced
1 tsp dried oregano
Salt & pepper to taste
Chopped green olives to serve (about 5 sliced per person)

In a large pan, fry onion and carrot in olive oil until the onion is translucent. Add garlic and stir for a couple of minutes, taking care not to burn. Add the mince and fry until brown. Add the cooked oregano and tomato puree and stir to coat the mince. Fry for 2-3 minutes. Add the chopped tomatoes and 1 tin of water. Add the mushrooms and seasoning.

Bring to the boil and simmer very gently for 30-60 minutes until the beef is tender and the sauce is thick. This works very well made the night before.

Try serving with courgetti and/or mixed salad for a low-carb alternative.

Or add 100g cooked pasta at 131 calories.

Chilli Con Carne

Serves 4: Approx. Calories per portion 450

This is another crowd-pleaser that works brilliantly without the traditional carbs.

1lb minced beef (Calories based on 15% fat mince, use lower fat if available/preferred)
1 onion chopped
1 green pepper chopped
15g olive oil
Clove garlic chopped
1 x tins tomatoes
1 x tin kidney beans
1 tbs tomato puree
Chilli powder to taste
1 tsp oregano
1tsp cumin (optional)
1 tsp vinegar
Salt & pepper
Chopped coriander to serve

In a large pan, fry onion and pepper until soft in the oil. Add the mince to the pan and fry until browned. Add the garlic and fry for a couple of minutes, then add chilli, cumin, oregano and vinegar and stir to combine. Add the tomato puree and fry for a few minutes stirring constantly to mix everything together. Add the tinned tomatoes and bring to the boil and simmer for 20 mins. Add kidney beans and simmer for a further 10 mins, until everything is cooked through, and the sauce is thickened. Check seasoning and serve sprinkled with chopped coriander.

Serving options:

Serve with mixed salad + 35 calories, 100g boiled rice +130 calories, 100g baked potato +93 calories.

Make it kid-friendly - arrange tortilla chips on a plate, spoon chilli over the top, top with grated cheese and put under the grill to melt.

Chilli Non-Carne

Replacing meat with pulses makes a satisfying and low-cost option.

Serves 4: Approx. calories per portion 375

1 onion chopped
1 green pepper chopped
1 red pepper chopped
15g olive oil
Clove garlic chopped
2 x tins tomatoes
1 x tin kidney beans
2 x tins green lentils
2 tbs tomato puree
Chilli powder to taste
1 tsp oregano
1tsp cumin (optional)
1 tsp vinegar
Salt & pepper
Chopped coriander to serve

In a large pan, fry onion and pepper in the oil until soft. Add garlic and fry for a couple of minutes, then add chilli, cumin, oregano and vinegar and fry for a couple of minutes. Add tomato puree and fry for a few minutes stirring constantly. Add tinned tomatoes and bring to the boil and simmer for 20 mins. Add kidney beans and tinned lentils and simmer for 10 mins, until reduced and the sauce is thick. Check seasoning and serve sprinkled with chopped coriander.

Serving options:

Serve with mixed salad + 35 calories, 100g boiled rice +130 calories, 100g baked potato +93 calories.

Make it kid-friendly - arrange tortilla chips on a plate, spoon chilli over the top, top with grated cheese and put under the grill to melt.

Lamb Donner Kebab & Yoghurt Sauce

Serves 4: Approx. calories per portion 440

Get all the taste of a favourite takeaway with fewer calories and none of the guilt. Lamb mince is very fatty, but the fat will drain out while it cooks. As soon as you take it out of the oven, lift the lamb loaf out of the tin, leaving the fat behind.

2 x 250g packs of minced lamb
2 cloves grated garlic
1 tbs chopped coriander
2 tsp cumin
2 tsp smoked paprika
1 tsp dried mint
Salt & pepper

Yoghurt Sauce. To make the yoghurt sauce, finely chop 1/3 cucumber and add to 150g Greek yoghurt. Add a squeeze of lemon, pinch of salt and 1/2 tsp chopped mint.

Marinated Onions. Finely slice one onion and marinate in a large pinch of salt and the juice of half a lemon. Leave for 20 minutes.

Mixed Salad. Mix sliced lettuce with chopped tomato and cucumber.

Mix the spices into the lamb and turn it into a loaf tin.

Bake in the oven at 180 degrees until piping hot and cooked through (30-40mins)

Drain off any excess fat and turn onto a chopping board Slice finely to resemble donner kebab. Serve with the salad, onions and yoghurt sauce.

Serving Options:

Add pitta bread + 145 calories or tortilla wrap +144

Calories may vary depending on size and brand, so check the packaging.

Cheese Burger & Sweet Potato Fries

Serves 1: Approx. calories 525

1 quarter pounder burger (or vegetarian/vegan alternative) 15g cheddar cheese
100g sweet potato sliced into thick batons
1 tsp coconut oil
Mixed salad (lettuce, cucumber, tomato)
1 tbs mayo (optional, or replace with oil and vinegar for salad)

Roast the sweet potato in the coconut oil until cooked and crispy (approx. 30mins). Bake the burger in the oven until cooked, and drain the fat (See packaging for timing). Add cheese to the burger and return to the oven for a couple of minutes until melted. Serve with the salad and a dollop of mayo.

Piri Piri Chicken with Slaw

A handy family recipe which is popular with the kids.

Serves 2: Approx. calories per serving 550

Chicken

2 medium chicken breasts (approx. 300g)
1 clove garlic grated
1/2 tsp chilli flakes (or to taste)
1 tsp smoked paprika
1/2 tsp dried oregano
1 tsp red wine vinegar
2 tsp olive oil
Salt & pepper

Dice the chicken and marinade in the other ingredients for at least 1 hour or overnight. To cook, preheat the oven to 180, place the chicken on a non-stick baking sheet and cook for approx. 25 minutes until cooked through and lightly brown. Serve with the slaw.

Slaw

300g summer cabbage
100g frozen peas, defrosted and cooked
50g sliced radish
1-2tbs fresh mint, chopped (or 1 tsp dried)
2tbs of mayo

Salt pepper to taste

Finely slice the cabbage and the radish. Season and add the mint. Mix in the mayo and stir well to combine.

Optional extras:

To keep the kids happy, serve with oven chips. Check packaging for calories.

Harissa Lamb Leg Steak with Tsatziki & Slaw

Serves 1: Approx. calories 480

Take 1 lamb leg steak and spread with 1-2 tsp of harissa paste from a jar (to taste) and leave to marinate for at least an hour or overnight.

Tzatziki

50g Greek yoghurt
10cms of cucumber grated
Salt
1/4 tsp dried mint
1 tsp olive oil
Lemon juice

Slaw

50g summer cabbage
Half a red pepper sliced
4 radishes sliced
1/2 lemon juiced
Salt & pepper
5ml olive oil

Place the marinated lamb on an oven tray and bake in the oven at 180 degrees for 20-25 minutes until cooked through. Grate the cucumber and sprinkle with a large pinch of salt. Leave for 5-10 minutes, then drain and squeeze dry. Add to the yoghurt, mint olive oil and lemon juice. Season to taste.

Finely slice the cabbage and mix with the pepper and radish. Add the lemon juice, salt, pepper and olive oil and mix. Leave for 10-15 minutes for the cabbage to soften slightly. When the lamb is cooked, serve with the salad and tzatziki.

Making Vegetables the Main Event

One of the main principles behind this eating programme is to replace low nutrient carbs (bread, pasta, rice, potatoes) with more nutritious carbs, like vegetables and pulses. As we age, we need more nutrients to build and repair tissues. The more nutritious we make our meals, the more support we give our body to keep our hormones balanced, which is vital from your 40s onwards.

If you are vegetarian or vegan, or just choosing to eat less meat, plan your meals around tasty vegetable dishes. Then, add your favourite protein and check you're eating enough protein to keep you full. Be wary of fake vegan meats, which are heavily processed. Check labels to ensure they include a reasonable amount of protein.

Vegetarian Protein Sources:

Cheese
Greek yoghurt
Eggs
Plus all vegan proteins

Vegan Protein Sources:

Tofu
Nuts
Seeds
Pulses
Legumes
Quinoa
Buckwheat
Chia seeds

Table of Protein in Foods

Use the following recipes to make a meal based on vegetables, then add protein of your choice to create a complete, filling meal. For vegetarians and vegans, combining more than one type of protein is recommended so you eat a wider range of essential amino acids.

Food	Serving Size	Total Calories	Protein g
Eggs	2 small (approx. 100g)	131	13g
Prawns	100g	99	24g
Cod fillet	100g	82	18g
Chicken breast	100g	165	31g
Steak	100g	271	25g
Minced beef 10% fat	100g	176	20g

Greek Yoghurt (0% fat)*	100g	59	10g
Natural Yogurt 3.3% fat*	100g	61	3.5g
Cheddar cheese	30g	121	7.5g
Feta cheese	50g	132	7g
Tofu	100g	76	8g
Buckwheat Grains	100g, boiled	118	4.3g
Quinoa	100g, boiled	120	4.4
Chia Seeds	50g	243	8.5g
Almonds	30g	188	8.7g
Tinned Green Lentils, Drained	100g	95	6g
Tinned Chickpeas, Drained	100g	119	5g
Green Peas	100g	81	5g
Edamame Beans, Frozen	100g	122	11g
Rolled oats*	50g	190	6.6g

*Check labels for individual nutrition.

Source USDA

Cauliflower & Broccoli Rice

Calories are shown for the total recipe. Simply divide the total based on what you are eating.

Total calories per recipe 324

300g cauliflower
300g broccoli
20ml olive oil
Salt and pepper to taste
Chopped coriander (optional)
Grated lemon rind (optional)

Chop the veg into chunks and process in a food processor until chopped into a fine rice-like texture. Heat the oil in a large frying pan on a medium heat and tip the riced veg into the pan.

Sauté, stirring regularly to coat the grains in the oil. Continue stirring until the grains are browned and cooked through, taking care not to burn them. If needed, add a splash of water to the pan.

When tender, season to taste and add extra herbs if using.

Beans, Lentils & Tomatoes

Calories are shown for the total recipe. Simply divide the total based on what you are eating.

Total calories per recipe 530

1 tin of brown or green lentils, drained and rinsed
80g frozen green beans
80g frozen peas
80g frozen broad beans
4 medium tomatoes, deseeded and chopped
1-2tbs of chopped herbs e.g. parsley, tarragon, mint, coriander.
1 tbs olive oil
Vinegar or lemon juice to taste
Salt & pepper to taste

Add tomato and herbs to a large bowl. Add frozen veg to a pan of boiling water and simmer until just tender; drain and add to the tomato mix. Add the lentils, the oil, vinegar or lemon and seasoning. Gently mix everything together and adjust seasoning to taste. Serve warm or cold.

Cauliflower, Broccoli, Lentils

Calories are shown for the total recipe. Simply divide the total based on what you are eating.

Total calories per recipe 543

1 small head of cauliflower sliced into small chunks
1 medium head of broccoli sliced into small florets
1 tin of brown or green lentils
1/2 finely sliced white or red onion, marinated in salt and lemon while the veg are roasting.
10g coconut oil (for roasting the veg) 1 tbs olive oil
Salt & pepper to taste

Heat the oven to 180 degrees. Put the coconut oil on a large baking tray and put it in the oven for a couple of minutes to melt. Tip the cauliflower and broccoli onto the tray and toss lightly to coat in the oil. Return to the oven for 20-25 minutes. Check them every 10 minutes to ensure they are not burning. If needed, give them a stir, so they cook evenly. Cooking time will depend on how small you chopped the veg. They are done when they are lightly charred and tender.

When they are done, mix with the rest of the ingredients, season to taste and serve warm or cold.

Courgette & Chickpeas

Calories are shown for the total recipe. Simply divide the total based on what you are eating.

Total calories per recipe 485

4 medium courgettes sliced
1 tin chickpeas
Juice and rind of a lemon
1 tbs olive oil
Salt & pepper to taste
1 tbs chopped coriander (optional)
2 tsp coconut oil

Heat the coconut oil on a griddle until smoking, and griddle the courgette in batches until charred on each side. Lay on a plate as they are done and season with salt, pepper and grated lemon rind Drain and rinse the chickpeas and mix with more lemon rind, olive oil, and lemon juice and season to taste. Sprinkle over the courgettes. Finish with the coriander if using. Serve warm or cold.

Roast Summer Vegetables

Calories are shown for the total recipe Simply divide the total based on what you are eating.

Total calories per recipe 119

1 red pepper chopped
1 yellow pepper chopped
2 medium red onions sliced into wedges
2 medium courgettes chopped into chunks
1 tbs olive oil
Chopped or dried herbs to garnish (optional), e.g. basil, oregano)

Heat the oven to 180 degrees. Put the coconut oil on a large baking tray and put in the oven for a couple of minutes to melt. Add the veg to the tray and stir to coat with the oil. Return to the oven for 20-25 minutes. Check them every 10 minutes or so to make sure they are not burning. Give them a stir if needed, so they cook evenly. Cooking time will depend on how small you chopped the veg.

Add tinned beans or pulses of your choice to make this more substantial and increase protein.

Cabbage Slaw

Calories are shown for the total recipe. Works well with red or white cabbage, the soft, inner leaves of savoy cabbage, or pointed summer cabbage.

Total calories per recipe 319

Half a head of cabbage (approx. 300g)
Half an onion sliced and marinated in lemon and salt for 10mins
1 carrot chopped into matchsticks
8 radishes sliced
80g frozen peas defrosted
1tbs olive oil & vinegar to taste (or 1tbs of mayo)
Salt and pepper to taste
2tbs chopped herbs, e.g. coriander, mint, parsley

Mix everything together and season to taste.

Spring Vegetables

Approx. calories per recipe 488

200g sprouting broccoli
200g asparagus spears
100g frozen broad beans, defrosted and cooked
100g peas, defrosted and cooked
Mint
Lemon rind and juice
15ml olive oil
30g shaved parmesan or pecorino cheese (optional)
Salt and pepper

Trim and cut the broccoli into similar-sized pieces. Trim the asparagus and cut in half. In a large saute pan with a lid, add the broccoli and a splash of water. Cover with the lid and steam for 2-3 minutes. Add the asparagus and steam for a further 2 minutes, adding another splash of water if needed. Add the peas and broad beans and cover for 2 minutes until warm. Drain off excess liquid. Add the mint, lemon rind and olive oil and mix. Season to taste and top with the parmesan or pecorino if using.

Autumn Vegetables

Approx. calories per recipe 776

400g butternut squash, peeled and diced into large cubes
2 red peppers
1 tin puy lentils drained and rinsed
15 ml olive oil
10ml olive oil for dressing & red wine vinegar
Salt and pepper

Place the butternut squash in a large roasting tray and toss in 15ml olive oil to coat. Roast at 180 degrees for 30-40minutes until evenly cooked. Allow to cool slightly. Tip the drained and rinsed lentils into a large bowl, season with more oil, a splash of red wine vinegar and salt and pepper. Add the cooked squash and mix gently. Adjust seasoning. Serve warm or cold.

Mushrooms, Lentils & Rocket

Approx. calories per recipe 452

200g button mushrooms, cleaned and sliced
2 cloves garlic
15ml olive oil
200g puy lentils drained and rinsed.
Couple of large handfuls of rocket or spinach
Salt & pepper

Heat the oil in a large frying pan and add the mushrooms, fry until soft Add the garlic and stir until cooked. Add the lentils into the pan and mix to warm through. Season to taste. Add the rocket or spinach and serve immediately. Serve warm or cold.

Warm red cabbage

Approx. calories per recipe 283

400g red cabbage, finely sliced
1 red onion, finely sliced
2 cloves garlic, finely chopped
15ml olive oil
Cinnamon stick
50-100ml water or stock

Heat the oil and add the onion and cook on a low heat until caramelised and meltingly soft, about 20 minutes. Stir occasionally to make sure it doesn't catch. Add the garlic and cinnamon stick and fry for a couple of minutes, then add the cabbage, stirring to coat in the oil and spices. Add about 50ml of water or stock, turn up the heat until the water boils, then turn right down and cover pan. Check regularly to stir and check the cabbage is not catching. The cabbage is ready when it's soft, and the liquid has reduced right down. Season to taste and remove the cinnamon stick. Best served warm.

Roast Winter Vegetables

Approx. calories per recipe 448

200g Carrots
200g Parsnips
200g Celeriac
2 Red onions
15ml olive oil
Salt & pepper

Peel and chop the vegetables into similar-sized pieces. Pour the oil into a roasting tin, add the veg and stir to coat. Place in a preheated oven at 180 degrees. Cook for 30-40 minutes, stirring occasionally.

Butterbean Mash

Approx. calories per recipe 520

Two tins of butterbeans, drained and rinsed, approx. 450g
15ml olive oil
2 cloves garlic finely chopped
Grated rind and juice of ½-1 lemon
Salt and pepper

Gently fry the garlic in the olive oil in a medium pan. When cooked but not brown, tip the butterbeans in and carefully mash them up, mixing them into the garlic and oil. Add lemon rind and half the juice of the lemon and briefly bring to the boil before turning down again, adding more lemon juice or water to taste. The liquid will help soften the beans, making them easier to mash. When the beans reach a mash-like consistency, add salt and pepper to taste and serve warm.

Mixed Salad

Chopping up a range of raw salad vegetables is quick and easy, and kids often prefer raw to cooked vegetables. They are a good source of fibre, and add bulk to meals which is important to replace the filling feeling you get from pasta and rice. For fussy kids (and adults), chop veg and place separately on a large plate so they can help themselves to the things they like.

A portion of 150g of mixed salad veggies is approx. 35 calories Choose from:

Lettuce
Cabbage
Tomatoes
Cucumber
Peppers
Radish
Courgette
Onion
Celery
Spring onion
Chopped herbs (coriander, mint, parsley, basil)

Optional dressings: 10ml olive oil = 80 calories 1tbs full fat mayo = 105, Vinegar, lemon, salt, pepper 0 calories

Hummus

Calories are shown for the total recipe. Simply divide the total based on what you are eating. Home-made hummus has fewer calories than shop-bought, which are also often made with lower quality oils.

Total calories per recipe 777

1 tin of chickpeas, drained and canning liquid reserved
2 tbs tahini
10ml olive oil
Juice of 1 lemon
Salt & pepper to taste
Paprika
1 tsp olive oil to garnish

Tip the chickpeas into a blender, reserving about a tablespoon for garnishing. Add the tahini, olive oil, lemon juice and seasoning and blend to a thick paste. Add about a tbs of water or reserved liquid to thin to your preferred consistency. Tip into a bowl and garnish with the reserved chickpeas, paprika and a drizzle of oil.

Tomato & Chilli Sauce

Total calories 140

1 clove garlic
10ml olive oil
Chilli flakes to taste
1 tsp smoked paprika
2 tbs tomato paste

Fry the garlic in the oil until translucent. Add the chilli flakes, paprika and tomato paste and fry in the oil for 2-3 minutes on a medium heat, taking care not to burn the garlic.

Add water and seasoning to get a medium-thin consistency.

Baba Ghanoush

Total calories: Approx. 423

1 medium aubergine
2 tbs tahini
Juice half a lemon
1 clove of garlic, grated
1 tbs olive oil
Salt & pepper to taste

Place the aubergine on a griddle and set over high heat. Turn the aubergine every 5-10 minutes until charred on the outside and completely softened and collapsed. Leave to cool slightly before removing the skin and scraping the soft flesh from the inside into a medium bowl. Grate over the garlic, add the tahini and lemon juice and mash to a smooth paste, adding more lemon or a splash of water if desired to loosen the texture. You can blend in a blender if you like, which will create a much smoother dip. Season to taste, drizzle over the oil and serve warm or cold.

Snack Ideas

Work to reduce the number of snacks you have and try and wean yourself off eating sweet snacks during the day. We mostly want to snack out of habit, rather than true hunger, although I notice that I have cravings when I've not eaten enough protein. When this happens, I eat something high protein, like a couple of scrambled eggs.

Two or three scrambled eggs in 5g butter

Hard-boiled eggs

Two or three oat cakes with a tablespoon of dip (see above), cottage cheese, or thinly-sliced hard cheese or cooked meat

Two or three oat cakes with a thin scraping of peanut butter

A small handful of nuts, around 25-30g

Frozen berries and a spoonful of Greek yoghurt (or sugar-free plant-based alternative)

A couple of spoonfuls of Greek yoghurt (or sugar-free plant-based alternative)with a tablespoon of mixed seeds or desiccated coconut

10-15 Black or Green Olives in brine

Sliced meat of choice with sliced vegetable crudites

A small tin of tuna mashed with a teaspoon of mayo with sliced vegetable crudites

Hummus, tzatziki or baba ganoush dip with sliced vegetable crudites

A couple of squares of dark chocolate (70% and above)

Making Your Own Meals

I encourage you to experiment with meals that work for you and your family. To put together a meal, follow this template.

Start with Protein

Protein keeps you full and makes meals satisfying. You can grill, stew or fry protein. When frying, use as little oil as possible. Marinating your protein adds taste and increases your enjoyment of meals. Use your favourite herbs and spices, mixed with a little oil or yoghurt and vinegar or lemon juice. Season and leave for a couple of hours before cooking.

Use the table overleaf as a guide to portion sizes, calories and protein content.

Add Unlimited Vegetables

Mix and match your favourite vegetables. You can serve vegetables raw or try grilling, frying in a little oil, boiling, or steaming. You can mix raw and cooked vegetables together. For example, I often roast peppers, courgettes and onions and add them to mixed salads.

Don't worry about portion sizes as most vegetables are very low calorie so pile your plate high.

Food	Serving Size	Total Calories	Protein g
Eggs	2 small (approx. 100g)	131	13g
Prawns	100g	99	24g
Cod fillet	100g	82	18g
Chicken breast	100g	165	31g
Steak	100g	271	25g
Minced beef 10% fat	100g	176	20g
Greek Yoghurt (0% fat)*	100g	59	10g
Natural Yogurt 3.3% fat*	100g	61	3.5g
Cheddar cheese	30g	121	7.5g
Feta cheese	50g	132	7g
Tofu	100g	76	8g
Buckwheat Grains	100g, boiled	118	4.3g
Quinoa	100g, boiled	120	4.4
Chia Seeds	50g	243	8.5g
Almonds	30g	188	8.7g

Tinned Green Lentils, Drained	100g	95	6g
Tinned Chickpeas, Drained	100g	119	5g
Green Peas	100g	81	5g
Edamame Beans, Frozen	100g	122	11g
Rolled oats*	50g	190	6.6g

*Check labels for individual nutrition.
Source USDA

Add Bulk with Pulses and Starchy Carbohydrates

Tinned lentils, chickpeas and beans are handy store cupboard staples. They are cheap and two or three tablespoons combine brilliantly with protein and vegetables to add bulk and texture.

If you enjoy rice, pasta, and potatoes with meals, feel free to add them but keep an eye on portion size. Follow these useful guidelines from the British Dietetic Association (BDA).

Cooked Pasta 2-3 tablespoons
Cooked Rice 2-3 tablespoons
New Potatoes 3 egg-sized or 6 thumb-sized
Baked Potatoes 1 medium (around 175g)
Porridge Oats 3 tablespoons

Make Tasty With Fat

A small amount of fat adds taste to many dishes. Add a small knob of butter to steamed vegetables or drizzle with a tablespoon of oil.

Avocados and olives are high fat vegetables which make a lovely addition to salads and vegetable dishes.

Coconut milk adds richness to curries and stews but is very high in calories so don't use too much. Check calories on the tins and measure out accurately.

Cheese is also a tasty addition to many dishes. Chop feta into salad, grate hard cheese into soups and onto roast vegetables or potatoes before putting under the grill to brown. Again, cheese is high calorie so aim for around 20g – 30g.

Add texture & taste

Herbs and spices add barely any calories, so use freely.

Chopped, toasted nuts and seeds add crunch. Use around a tablespoon so you don't add too many calories.

Raw veg can also liven up salads and vegetables, try adding thinly sliced onions or spring onions. You can marinate them in a little lemon juice and salt for half an hour to reduce the strong taste.

Combine different vegetables together to add interest and texture.

Check the Calories

You can add your own recipes into MyFitnessPal or similar apps, so you can check how many calories your creations have.

Beginners' Strength Programme

Get Strong in One Hour

Is it even possible to get stronger in one hour? Yes, it is. I've trained many 40+ women who only did one hour of strength training a week, and they measurably improved their strength. If you are new to exercise or have got out of the habit, doing an hour a week is plenty, and you'll quickly feel the benefits.

The main reason to aim for one hour is that it's achievable and effective. This programme has been written for stressed, busy women who don't have much time. By starting with something realistic, there's less pressure, and you're more likely to succeed. It's just enough for you to notice the benefits whilst avoiding the discomfort and exhaustion of overdoing it.

This easy and effective strength programme won't leave you feeling sore and exhausted. It targets all the major muscles in your body to give you a balanced workout, and you'll feel energised afterwards. Don't be tempted to do more than this, to begin with. Instead, prioritise building consistency because you'll only get the benefits of exercise if you do it regularly.

You're going to do two 30-minute sessions of strength training a week for 4 weeks. Leave 2 to 4 days between sessions to allow your body to recover. It's essential to use the correct technique for each exercise. If you've not done these exercises before or are a bit rusty, watch the instruction videos I've created for you. See below for details of how to find them.

Before You Start

Before starting a new diet or exercise programme, you must visit your GP first. This is especially important if you have an existing medical condition, take any medication, have recently suffered injuries, or had any operations in the past few months. If you've not had your blood pressure taken recently, then get this checked before you start exercising. Exercising is safe for most people, but it's vital to ensure you are in good health before you begin. Your doctor must confirm that it won't worsen your condition or alter medication doses. Do not work out on your own if you have low blood pressure, poor balance, or suffer from fainting or blackouts. When you exercise, if you begin to feel unwell in any way, stop immediately and seek urgent medical advice.

The Equipment

I recommend investing in a few key pieces of equipment to get the best results from your workouts. I promise they won't take up much room, but they will make your workouts more effective.

Choosing the right weight

I recommend buying a pair of dumbbells in 2kg, 3kg and 5kg weights. The lighter weights are mainly for arm exercises and the heavier ones for leg exercises. To begin with, use the lightest weight for each exercise. If you can repeat the exercise 12 times and it feels easy, the weight is too light, so choose a heavier one. You'll know you're using the right weight when you can perform 8-10 repetitions of an exercise, but the last 2 or 3 feel difficult, and you need a short rest when you've finished.

After a few weeks of performing these exercises, they will start to feel easier. When you can comfortably do 12 reps, it's time to increase the weight.

Equipment	Used For	Good Places to Buy From	Link to Websites
Dumbbell (Pairs) Start with 2kg, 3kg, 5kg	Arm & shoulder exercises Squats & lunges	Decathlon Argos Mirafit	https://www.decathlon.co.uk/browse/c0-sports/c1-fitness-and-gym/c3-dumbbells/_/N-12fopdnZo6kh17 https://www.argos.co.uk/search/dumbbells/type:dumbbells/ https://mirafit.co.uk/weights-and-bars/dumbbells.html
Glute Bands	Various glute exercises	Decathlon BC Strength	https://www.decathlon.co.uk/search?Ntt=glute+band https://www.bcstrength.co.uk/collections/resistance-bands
Exercise Bands	Pulling exercises	Decathlon	https://www.decathlon.co.uk/p/cross-training-elastic-training-band-5-kg/_/R-p-307521?mc=8552664&c=BLUE

Adjustable Step* *Check the step that you buy is suitable for your current body weight	Step up lunges, Glute exercises, Chest exercises	Decathlon Powerhouse Fitness	https://www.decathlon.co.uk/search?Ntt=training+step https://www.powerhouse-fitness.co.uk/fitness-accessories/fitness-steps
Exercise Mat	All exercises to prevent slipping	Decathlon	https://www.decathlon.co.uk/search?Ntt=exercise+mat

Correct form

The most important part of strength training is to follow the correct technique. You'll get the best results and reduce your chance of getting injured. Watch the videos for each exercise first. It may take longer to begin with while you get the hang of them. If you aren't sure you're doing them right, book a couple of sessions with a personal trainer so they can show you. Some personal trainers will come to your house, others work from private gyms. To find a qualified trainer in your area, use this link:

https://www.cimspa.co.uk/directories

Click on the browse members button to find qualified and registered personal trainers.

Reps & Sets

Reps: Exercises are repeated 8 - 12 times; therefore, you do 8-12 reps

Sets: When you have completed your reps, you have done one set.

For example, these are the instructions for one of the exercises:

Exercise	Equipment	Reps	Sets
Shoulder press	Dumbbells	8 - 12	2 or 3

A shoulder press is an exercise involving raising dumbbells over your head to strengthen the shoulder muscles. I've suggested you repeat this exercise 8 or 12 times (the reps). Do as many as it takes for the last 2 or 3 reps to feel challenging but doable. To begin with, you may only be able to do 8 reps before it feels too hard. After a few sessions, you might be able to get to 12. After you have done your first set, have a short rest before starting the next set.

You perform each exercise 3 times in total. If that's too much, start with 2 sets. As you become familiar with the routines and become stronger, increase the sets.

Warm up & Stretching

Each workout includes a warm-up and stretches at the end. Don't skip this, as it helps avoid injuries and tight muscles. It's common for muscles to ache around 24 to 48 hours after exercise, particularly when you start a new regime. To ease aching muscles, drink plenty of water, keep moving and do light stretches. Warm baths help, especially with added magnesium salts. Once you've got used to exercising you won't suffer as much.

When to Stop Exercising

Stop immediately if you feel dizzy, faint, experience chest pains, pain in your arms, or feel unwell in any way and call emergency services. If you feel any sudden, sharp pain when exercising, stop. Pain from injury is different from the feeling of discomfort from muscles being worked. The latter feels like an ache that develops gradually in the muscles as they become tired. Pulled muscles and sprains are sharper and more sudden. Don't ignore these feelings. Likewise, stop if you feel any sharp or persistent pains in your joints. If you think you've pulled a muscle or sprained a joint, seek help from your doctor or physiotherapist or call the emergency services if you're worried.

Regardless of whether we exercise or not, most people will suffer from sprains and strains now and again. In the long term, exercise will make you stronger, less likely to suffer from these issues and able to recover faster if you do.

The Workouts

I have given you two 30 minutes workouts. One for the upper body, and one for the lower body. Both workouts include stomach exercises.

Workout One - Upper Body

Exercise	Equipment	Reps	Sets
Warm-up	-	-	-
Row (with band)	5kg band	8 - 12	2 or 3
Shoulder press	Dumbbells	8 - 12	2 or 3
Chest press	Step or floor Dumbbells	8 - 12	2 or 3
Tricep press	Dumbbells	8 - 12	2 or 3
Bicep curl	Dumbbells	8 - 12	2 or 3
Sidearm raise	Dumbbells	8 - 12	2 or 3
Side bend	Dumbbells	8 – 12	2 or 3
Ab crunch	Bodyweight or dumbbells	8 – 12	2 or 3
Toe Taps	Bodyweight or dumbbells	8 – 12	2 or 3
Oblique crunch	Bodyweight	8 – 12	2 or 3
Back Extension	Bodyweight	8 – 12	2 or 3
Stretches	-	-	-

Workout Two - Lower Body

Exercise	Equipment	Reps	Sets
Warm-up	-	-	-
Squat (sit to stand)	Bodyweight or dumbbells of your choice	8 – 12	2 or 3
Step up lunge	Step, Bodyweight or dumbbells of your choice	8 – 12	2 or 3
Glute Bridge	Bodyweight or band	8 – 12	2 or 3

Side-Lying Leg Raise	Bodyweight or band	8 – 12	2 or 3
Clamshells	Bodyweight	8 – 12	2 or 3
Straight arm plank	Bodyweight	8 – 12	2 or 3
Deadbug	Bodyweight	8 – 12	2 or 3
Side Plank	Bodyweight	8 – 12	2 or 3
Back Extension	Bodyweight	8 – 12	2 or 3
Stretches	-	-	-

Exercise Videos & Bonus Workouts

I've set up a dedicated page on my website with all exercise and workout videos. You'll also find bonus workouts, so you can vary the sessions as you progress. For days when you are pushed for time, there are some 15 and 20-minute sessions too.

You can find all the exercise videos on www.gabrielleohare.com/book-resources

Free Resources

Readers also have access to the following resources on www.gabrielleohare.com/book-resources

Free Facebook support group

New Recipes

Bonus Workouts

Guided breathwork and meditation techniques

REFERENCES

(1) Cortisol and its link to increased abdominal fat
https://pubmed.ncbi.nlm.nih.gov/16353426/

(2) Effect of poor sleep on eating habits
https://www.ncbi.nlm.nih.gov/pmc/articles/PMC3763921/

(3) NHS Menopause Average age and symptoms
https://www.nhs.uk/conditions/menopause/symptoms/

(4) Age related muscle loss. Source Ageless: The New Science of Getting Older Without Getting Old by Andrew Steele.

(5) Muscle loss after menopause
https://www.ncbi.nlm.nih.gov/pmc/articles/PMC7956097/

(6) Early retirement due to menopause. Survey by Newson Health Research and Education.

(7) Obesity rates in older adults.
https://researchbriefings.files.parliament.uk/documents/SN03336/SN03336.pdf

(8) Percentage of calories from ultra-processed foods
https://www.bbc.co.uk/food/articles/what_is_ultra-processed_food#:~:text=Issues%20arise%20when%20ultra%2Dprocessed,come%20from%20ultra%2Dprocessed%20foods

(9) Amount of ultra-processed food in shopping https://www.soilassociation.org/media/21669/ultra-processed-foods_soil-association-report.pdf

(10) Percentage of food in supermarkets falling into ultra-processed category https://bmjopen.bmj.com/content/9/10/e027546

(11) Men have more ability than women to control their brain's response to their favourite foods. https://www.bnl.gov/newsroom/news.php?a=110876

(12) Women's hunger hormones rise faster than mens after eating https://academic.oup.com/jcem/article/98/5/E847/2537151

(13) Ultra-processed foods and weight gain. https://www.health.harvard.edu/blog/what-are-ultra-processed-foods-and-are-they-bad-for-our-health-2020010918605

(14) Effect on health of eating too much sugar https://www.medicalnewstoday.com/articles/eating-too-much-sugar

(15) Link between sugar consumption and depression https://www.ncbi.nlm.nih.gov/pmc/articles/PMC5532289/

(16) Link between sugar and joint pain https://www.webmd.com/rheumatoid-arthritis/features/sugar-ra-link

(17) Protein for Post Menopausal Women (ref: https://blog.nasm.org/protein-for-post-menopausal-women)

(18) Muscle loss during dieting
[https://www.ncbi.nlm.nih.gov/pmc/articles/PMC5421125/]

(19) Muscle gain for post-menopausal women who weren't taking HRT - Strong Women Stay Young' by Doctor Miriam E. Nelson, PhD.

(20) Exercise and Mental Health (*Source:
https://www.mentalhealth.org.uk/publications/how-to-using-exercise?gclid=Cj0KCQjw3v6SBhCsARIsACyrRAle6oYUr4G3E10
8tKX-
X547My80s34TVqLUCKzM2tAxFxT9jBYNV_oaAmWuEALw_
wcB)

(21) Lack of sleep and increase in dementia [https://www.nih.gov/news-events/nih-research-matters/lack-sleep-middle-age-may-increase-dementia-
risk#:~:text=People%20who%20slept%20six%20hours,importance
%20of%20good%20sleep%20habits]

Available worldwide online
and from all good bookstores

Michael Terence Publishing

www.mtp.agency

www.facebook.com/mtp.agency

@mtp_agency

Printed in Great Britain
by Amazon

16955839R00147